Natural Treatments for

ADD

and

HYPERACTIVITY

Natural Treatments for

ADD

and

HYPERACTIVITY

Skye Weintraub, N.D.

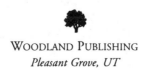

WOODLAND PUBLISHING
Pleasant Grove, UT

© 1997
Woodland Publishing, Inc.
P.O. Box 160
Pleasant Grove, UT
84062

TABLE OF CONTENTS

SECTION FOUR

WHAT ELSE? OTHER POSSIBLE CAUSES OF ADD

SECTION 5

TREATING ADD

Section One

UNDERSTANDING

ADD

Chapter 1

WHAT IS ADD?

INTRODUCTION

Can you imagine what it would be to live inside a fast-moving kaleidoscope? Sounds, images, color and movement—everything constantly shifting, constantly distracting you—your mind flitting and wandering because of the stimuli bombarding you. You would probably have trouble controlling yourself enough to concentrate and complete a task. Your mind would continuously be moving, so many things going on inside your head that sometimes you probably wouldn't even notice when someone was speaking to you.

This is what life is like for many children who have ADD. These kids seem to exist in a whirlwind of disorganized or frenzied activity. They are often unable to sit still and finish tasks, and at times are not fully aware of what is going on around them. But other times they seem fine. Periods of "normal" behavior lead people to assume that these children have control over their behavior, when really, that is not the case. Because of its erratic and difficult symptoms, ADD affects children's relationships with other people and is certainly very disruptive to their daily life. Children with ADD that are also hyperactive are not only extremely active, but can be demanding and interfering, particularly those who are elementary school age.

One of the difficulties with ADD is that parents may not even realize their child is exhibiting symptoms of the disorder. Parents who assume their child is healthy would be distressed to receive a note from school saying their child won't listen to the teacher, or that he is causing trouble in class. Because home life is very different from school, many parents do not see their child in certain situations. It is school, when the child has to maintain attention for long periods of time and is required to sit quietly, that problems can become quite evident. The impulsive behavior and inability to pay proper attention associated with ADD interfere with learning. Teachers, parents, and friends recognize that the child is "misbehaving," but they are often unable to tell exactly what is wrong.

Before 1980 the condition we now call attention deficit disorder was considered to be neurologically based. Physicians described the condition as "minimal brain dysfunction," despite the fact that the nature of the dysfunction remained unknown. By 1980, this clinical picture was renamed attention deficit disorder with hyperactivity or hyperkinesia. The American Psychiatric Association (APA) further subcategorized this problem into three subgroups: ADD with hyperactivity; ADD without hyperactivity; and ADD residual for adolescents. The definition of ADD has been further refined into three types: 1) predominantly inattentive, 2) predominantly hyperactive/impulsive, or 3) a combined type.

For the purpose of this book, attention deficit disorder (ADD) and attention deficit hyperactivity disorder (ADHD), a combination of hyperactivity and attention deficit disorder, will both be discussed under the title of ADD. These syndromes are usually discussed separately, but because much of this book discusses why people have these syndromes, it is important to recognize that the factors causing one may be equally relevant to the other.

A GENERAL DISCUSSION OF ADD AND HYPERACTIVITY

Hyperactivity often begins in the womb. Some mothers describe their children as "punching their way out of the uterus." Hyperactivity in infants manifests itself through head banging, crib rocking, colic, prolonged bouts of crying and screaming, general restlessness, great thirst, copious saliva and dribbling, and either fitful sleep or little need of sleep. Hyperactive babies are often difficult to feed and pacify, they resist affection and touch, and they have frequent tantrums. Another thing is that these infants are often slow to crawl.

As toddlers these same children are excitable, cry easily, and continue to burst into tantrums if their demands are not instantly met. They cannot sit still or concentrate on anything for more than a few seconds. They seem to be running everywhere and climbing on everything. It's hard to keep up with them because they are always on the move, touching everything and anything in reach, often breaking or destroying whatever they come in contact with. Sometimes, these kids turn their destructiveness on themselves, and this can be dangerous because they often seem to have a high pain threshold. A hyperactive toddler may bump into so many walls and pieces of furniture that it looks as if the parents are battering the child.

Many parents see signs of ADD in toddlers long before the children enter school. These children lose interest and dart off, even during their favorite TV shows or while playing games. Because children mature at different rates, and are very different in personality, temperament, and energy levels, it is useful to get an expert's opinion on whether certain behaviors are appropriate for a child's age. Parents often ask their pediatrician to assess whether their toddler has an attention disorder or is immature, hyperactive, or just exuberant.

By the time children with ADD reach first grade the symptoms appear to get even worse. In the classroom they do not seem to hear the teacher's instructions. They are easily distracted, make careless and impulsive errors, fail to follow through on requests, and feel socially isolated from their peers. These children cannot play games for the same amount of time as other children their age. They forget to write down school assignments or they take the wrong books home. As a result, homework is rarely finished or, if it does get done, it is usually full of mistakes. Children with ADD may have a normal or high IQ, but because of how the disorder affects them, they often still fail at school.

At home, other symptoms of ADD might be not being able to listen to a complete story, sit through a meal, or sleep through the night. Many children with ADD cannot complete a chore or follow directions and are unable to accept correction or discipline. These kids are too impulsive and usually do not think before they act. As a result, they do things like blurt out inappropriate comments or run into the street without looking. It is hard for them to wait for things they want or to take turns in a game. They are more likely to grab a toy from another child or hit others when upset. Their activities often lack direction or purpose. From these general descriptions, it is easy to see that ADD is not just an attention disorder, but a disorder of impulse control. Children with ADD actually do the things that other kids only think about. Their urge to act is not being inhibited, so their first reaction becomes their immediate behavior.

As these children grow they experience more difficulty in starting and completing tasks, making transitions, interacting with others, following through on directions, producing work consistently, and organizing multi-step tasks. Their actions are haphazard, poorly organized and not goal-oriented. New and different stimuli seem to attract their attention, and distractions may change with the moment. Difficulties arise when distractions are not considered important by a parent or teacher.

Other symptoms of ADD may also begin to manifest. These could include clumsiness, fatigue, listlessness, muscle weakness, body aches, aggression, nonstop talking, increased volume of speech, poor appetite, nervousness and anxiety, defiance and disobedience, depression, wild mood swings, high sensitivity to the environment, bed wetting, poor eye-hand coordination, swollen neck glands, fluid behind the ear drum, ringing in the ears, excessive sweating, dark eye circles or puffiness below the eyes, and self-abuse such as hair pulling.

It is important to realize that ADD is not a specific learning disability. Children with ADD have difficulty performing in school due to poor organization, impulsivity, and inattention. They are not unable to learn, but simply unavailable to learn. These children do not routinely show signs of serious emotional disturbance, but may develop problems with low self-esteem if the disorder is not properly treated. By the time they become adolescents, they often appear to be less hyperactive, but may still have many of the symptoms of ADD. Because of their poor learning skills and under-developed social skills, they continue to do poorly in school.

How Common is ADD?

During the 1950s and 1960s it would have been difficult to find children you could label with ADD. Today, however, you can find them in every school and in every classroom. One child out of every five suffers from a varying degrees of behavior problems. There is an explosion of disorders in school-age children today. These disorders involve learning difficulties experienced by children who would otherwise be considered intelligent and well-behaved.

It is interesting to note that there is a substantially greater incidence of ADD in boys than girls. As many as ten times more boys are diagnosed with ADD than girls. This may be because girls are less hyperactive and less likely to be diagnosed. Blond-haired and blue-eyed boys predominantly have ADD.

Onset of ADD is usually by the age of three, but the diagnosis is generally made when the child enters school. Twenty to thirty percent of the children diagnosed with ADD also have other learning disabilities, and 30 percent have delayed motor skill development. ADD is quickly becoming one of the most common health disorders today. It may now affect up to 20 percent of children in the American school system. It is the leading cause of failure in school for millions of kids. ADD often continues into adolescence and adulthood causing a lifetime of frustrated dreams and emotional pain.

HOW IS ADD DIAGNOSED?

There are no clear signs of ADD discernible on x-rays or lab tests. It is only certain characteristic behaviors that identify this condition, and these behaviors vary from child to child. There does not seem to be a single cause, but rather many possible causes. More than likely, ADD is simply a catch-all term for several slightly different disorders. At present, ADD is used as a diagnosis for children who consistently display certain characteristic behaviors over a period of time. The most common behaviors fall into three categories: inattention, hyperactivity, and impulsive behavior.

If you have questions or concerns regarding your child and ADD, begin by requesting an evaluation from your child's school. Seek further diagnostic assessment from trained professionals familiar with the condition. The best diagnostic process involves reports from the parents, teacher's observations, and a good, extensive family history which includes the child's developmental and medical history from birth. ADD should be diagnosed by the accumulation of information and the observation of behavior and performance of the child. Rule out all other possible sources before conceding to a diagnosis of ADD. A doctor should first look for and treat any other causes that could account for any ADD-like behaviors.

By the time there is a diagnosis, children with ADD have usually developed social or psychological problems. It is often helpful to seek counseling for both the child and the family. That way esteem issues or other problematic behaviors can be dealt with in a positive way. It is also helpful to obtain professional guidance in understanding and managing ADD.

BEHAVIOR PROFILE

Use the following questions to piece together a child's behavior profile. Your answers will help identify whether a child's hyperactivity, impulsivity, and inattention are significant and long-standing. If so, the child may be diagnosed with ADD.

- Which ADD-like behaviors listed in the Health Appraisal Questionnaire does your child have?
- How often does your child have these undesirable behaviors?
- In what situations?
- How old was the child when the problems started?
- Are the behaviors seriously interfering with your child's friendships, school activities, or home life?
- Does the child have any other related problems?

WHO MAKES THE DIAGNOSIS OF ADD?

School-age and preschool children are often evaluated by a school psychologist or a designated team of people. If the school doesn't believe the student has a problem, or if the family wants another opinion, a doctor in private practice should be consulted.

HOW DO SOME PROFESSIONALS DIAGNOSE ADD?

Professionals trained in the diagnosis of ADD compare a child's pattern of behavior against the set criteria and characteristics of the disorder. The current diagnostic criterion for ADD used by the American Psychiatric Association (APA) appears in the *Diagnostic and Statistical Manual of Mental Disorders* .

There are several other written tests available to diagnose children with ADD. Some of the rating scales used in assessing the disorder are: Conner's Teacher Rating Scale; ADD-H Comprehensive Teacher Rating Scale; ADHD Rating Scale; Child Attention Profile; Child Behavior Checklist; Home Situations Questionnaire; School Situations Questionnaire; and Academic Performance Rating Scale. One of the most popular assessment scales is the Conner's Parent

Rating Scale. Parents can rate children from ages three to seventeen using a 48-item questionnaire that covers five areas of assessment: conduct problems, learning disability, psychosomatic problems, impassivity, hyperactivity, and anxiety.

A TEAM APPROACH

A comprehensive assessment by a team of professionals working together can usually determine whether a child's problems are the result of ADD or other factors. Members of this assessment team would usually include physicians, psychologists, social workers, and school personnel such as teachers, guidance counselors, or learning specialists. Of course, also included are the parents and the child.

THE PHYSICIAN'S ROLE

When a decision has been made to explore the reasons for a child's ADD-like symptoms, the family can start by talking with the child's doctor or their family doctor. Some doctors do the assessment themselves, but more often they refer the family to a specialist. In addition, state and local agencies that serve families and children, as well as some volunteer organizations, may have facilities for testing.

As part of the assessment team the doctor needs to interview the child's teachers, parents, and other people who know the child well, such as school staff and baby-sitters. Gathering information can rule out other possible reasons for the child's behavior. The child's school and medical records will need to be checked. It is important to evaluate whether the home and classroom environments are stressful or chaotic, and how the child's parents and teachers deal with the child. Other medical conditions such as emotional disorders, undetectable seizures, and poor vision or hearing need to be ruled out. Most schools automatically screen for vision and hearing, but it is usually not adequate to detect some disorders. A doctor should also look at the child's diet, screen for allergies, evaluate nutritional levels, and test for metabolic disorders.

Because the doctor will play a huge role in your child's assessment, you need to choose your physician carefully. It is important to find someone with training and experience not only in diagnosing and treating ADD, but also other learning disabilities and developmental disorders. It is recommended that you find a doctor trained in natural healing. The reason for this is that the primary goal of naturopathic physicians is to look for the cause of the problem rather than simply treating the diagnosis of ADD. Their evaluation will be more holistic—they will investigate the possibilities of diet and nutritional deficiencies and excesses, heavy metal toxins, allergies and sensitivities, and more. Your child will receive a diagnosis that not only is complete, but one that will shed light on the factors that are the real root of your child's problems.

THE PSYCHOLOGIST'S ROLE

Clinical or school psychologists administer and interpret psychological and educational tests to guage things such as intelligence, attention span, visual-motor skills, memory, impulsivity, and language development. They also give tests to measure levels of achievement, and social and emotional adjustment. As part of a child's assessment team, psychologists and other mental health professionals often interpret data collected from behavior rating scales about the child in question. The information comes from people like the child's parents and teachers. Information may also be gathered about the child's ongoing behavior in order to compare it to the symptoms and diagnostic criteria listed in the *Diagnostic and Statistical Manual of Mental Disorders*. The psychologist needs to spend time talking with the child, and if possible, observe the child in the classroom and in other settings.

THE SCHOOL'S ROLE

Assessments of ADD should always include information about the student's current and past classroom performance, academic skills, strengths and weaknesses, attention span, and other social, emotional, or behavioral characteristics. The school can gather this information through teacher interviews, a review of cumulative records, analysis of test scores by a psychologist, and direct observation of the student in class. The school also needs to look at the student's curriculum, teacher expectations for the class and for the individual student, methods of instruction used by the teacher, incentives for finishing classwork, methods of teacher feedback to students, and comparative performance of other students in the class.

THE TEACHER'S ROLE

The teacher is often the first to recognize that a child has ADD and may consult with the school psychologist. Teachers work with many children so they know how the "average" child behaves in learning situations that require attention and self-control. However, teachers sometimes fail to notice the needs of children who are quiet and cooperative. The child's teachers, past and present, should rate the child's behavior using standardized evaluation forms. As always, any other type of learning disability needs to be ruled out.

THE CHILD'S ROLE

An interview with the child offers the opportunity to observe the child's behavior. It can yield valuable information about the child's social and emotional adjustment, feelings about themselves and others, attitudes about school, and other aspects of their life. Realize that the observations of a child's behavior when being interviewed may not be the same as when the child is in other settings. It has been found that children with ADD often behave normally in a one-on-one setting.

THE PARENTS' ROLE

Parents have the unique perspective of witnessing their child in a variety of situations over a number of years. Through interviews and questionnaires parents can inform the assessment team about their child. The focus is usually on obtaining an overall family history, as well as understanding the current family structure and function.

Important events from the child's medical, social, and academic history relevant to the assessment of ADD should be documented.

Parents will need to identify and describe their child's behavior in a variety of situations. They may also fill out a rating scale to indicate how severe and frequent the behaviors seem to be. How does the child behave during noisy or unstructured situations like parties? How does he perform during tasks that require sustained attention such as reading, working math problems, or playing a board game? Some parents may find it hard to see their child's behavior as a problem because it so closely resembles their own. These parents recognize that they too have ADD only when their child is diagnosed.

Labeling a child with ADD merely signifies that the child is displaying certain behavioral symptoms. The National Institutes of Health (NIH) says that the cluster of symptoms making up ADD does not represent a single disease, nor is it likely that the cause is singular; rather, the syndrome may be due to several causes. With a good assessment parents will be able to unravel the reasons their child has certain problems. Once the reasons become clear, a combination of educational, medical, and emotional help can be given. An effective treatment plan helps people with ADD and their families at many levels.

THE TEAM'S ROLE AFTER ASSESSMENT

Ideally, members of the assessment team should collaborate and discuss their findings during and after the process of data collection. This will lead to a thorough understanding of the child's strengths in areas of physical, academic, behavioral, and emotional needs. If there turns out to be a diagnosis of ADD (and/or other conditions), treatment planning can begin in all areas where recommended. The child's physician may discuss appropriate medical interventions with the child and parents. The psychologist, or other mental health professional, may discuss counseling, behavior modification, or social and organizational skills. The school may set up classroom interventions to accommodate the child's areas of need, or may provide special education and related services.

Once there is a completed assessment and proper medical treatment, there should be routine follow-ups by members of the team to determine how the child is progressing. ADD often requires long-term care and monitoring on a regular basis. Obviously, parents play a key role in encouraging members of the team to work together for the best interest of the child. Coordination of all this work, whether it be by a parent or a professional, is no easy task, but of course the outcome is usually well worth the effort.

EDUCATIONAL OPTIONS FOR CHILDREN WITH ADD

Children with ADD have a variety of needs. Some children are too hyperactive or inattentive to function in a regular classroom, even with medication and a behavior management plan. These children may function best in a special education class for all or part of the day. In some schools, the special education teacher teams up with the classroom teacher to meet each child's unique needs. However, most children are able to stay in the regular classroom. Whenever possible, educators prefer not to segregate children, but to let them learn along with their peers.

Although parents have the option of taking their child to a private practitioner for evaluation and educational services, most children with ADD qualify for free services within the public schools. Each child is entitled to receive an education that meets his or her unique needs. For example, the special education teacher working with parents, the school psychologist, school administrators, and the classroom teacher must assess the child's strengths and weaknesses and design an "individualized educational program," or IEP. The IEP outlines the specific skills the child needs to develop, as well as appropriate learning activities that build on the child's strengths. Parents play an important role in the process. They must be included in meetings and given an opportunity to review and approve their child's IEP.

Many children with ADD or other disabilities are also able to receive special education services under the Individuals with Disabilities Education Act (IDEA). The act guarantees appropriate services and a public education to children with disabilities from ages three to twenty-one. Those who do not qualify for services under IDEA can receive help under an earlier law, the National Rehabilitation Act, Section 504, which defines disabilities more broadly.

CAN OTHER DISORDERS ACCOMPANY ADD?

There are other problems that can accompany ADD—usually specific learning disabilities. A child will have trouble mastering language or certain other academic skills, typically reading and math. Also, nearly half of all children with ADD (mostly boys) tend to have another condition called "oppositional defiant disorder." These children may overreact or lash out when they feel bad about themselves. They may be stubborn, have outbursts of temper, or act belligerent or defiant. Sometimes this progresses to more serious conduct disorders. Children with this combination of problems are at risk of getting in trouble at school, and even with the law. They may steal, set fires, destroy property, drive recklessly, and take all kinds of risks. It is important that these children receive help before the behaviors lead to serious problems.

At some point, many children with ADD experience other emotional disorders. They feel anxious, worried, tense, or uneasy. This can affect their thinking and behavior. Some children experience depression which can disrupt sleep, appetite, and the ability to think. Having adults around who understand will help the children cope.

CAN ADD BE OUTGROWN
OR CURED?

Without finding the underlying cause of the symptoms, most people don't outgrow ADD. They just learn to adapt. Half of all children with ADD still show signs of the problem into adulthood. It is reassuring to know that children with ADD can usually develop normally if they have a treatment plan that includes a proper diet, nutritional balance, a decrease in the total toxic load to the body, a correction of any hearing and visual problems, treatment of any metabolic conditions, new training skills and emotional support. If children can develop certain skills, they can achieve personal goals. They may need to channel their excess energy into sports and other highly energetic activities. It is important to identify options that build on their strengths and abilities.

THE LONG-TERM PROGNOSIS

Approximately 80 percent of children with ADD will still meet the criteria for this diagnosis when adolescents. Most of them usually go on to become adults with ADD. This is why it is so important to find out what is causing your child's problem. There are numerous avenues to explore other than simply putting your child on a drug that will suppress the symptoms of ADD. The information in this book can be very helpful because it discusses myriad possible causes for ADD-like behavior.

Chapter 2

⌐⌐

A Health Appraisal

In order to ascertain whether your child is suffering from ADD or some other health problem, it is helpful to pinpoint certain behaviors and their possible causes. In my years as a physician, I have created the following questionnaire to serve as a guideline to help parents determine what is possibly wrong with their child and why. I also include the American Psychiatric Association's questionnaire to provide the criteria they use to determine whether or not a child has ADD.

CAN YOU DETERMINE IF YOUR CHILD HAS ADD?

The symptoms and causes of ADD-like behavior are extremely varied, so I have constructed a comprehensive list which includes those most commonly encountered. Read through the list and write "yes" next to the phrases that describe your child or your child's situation.

1. INATTENTION AND DISTRACTION

• has short attention span, especially for low-interest activities
• has difficulty or failure completing tasks or assignments; goofs off

- daydreams
- is easily distracted
- engages in much activity but accomplishes little
- does not listen when spoken to

2. IMPULSIVENESS

- acts before thinking
- is disorganized
- has poor planning ability
- often shifts from one activity to another
- has difficulty in group situations that require patience/taking turns
- requires much supervision
- is constantly in trouble
- frequently interrupts conversation & talks out of turn
- makes funny noises at inappropriate times

3. OVERACTIVITY OR HYPERACTIVITY

- is restless, fidgety or constantly on the go
- talks excessively
- excessive running, jumping, and climbing
- has difficulty staying seated or jumping up in class
- touches everything
- is easily excited

4. NON-COMPLIANCE

- frequently disobeys
- is argumentative
- disregards socially accepted standards of behavior

5. ATTENTION-GETTING BEHAVIOR

- frequently needs to be the center of attention
- constantly asks questions or interrupts
- irritates and annoys peers and adults
- is the "class clown"
- uses bad or rude language to attract attention
- engages in other negative behaviors to attract attention

6. IMMATURITY

- behavior resembles that of a child six months to two years younger
- physical development is delayed
- prefers to play with younger children and relates better to them
- has immature emotional reactions

7. UNDERACHIEVEMENT OR VISUAL-MOTOR PROBLEMS

- is an underachiever
- loses books, assignments, etc.
- has auditory processing problems
- has learning disabilities or learning problems
- does sloppy written work
- has poor memory for directions, instructions, and rote learning
- has vision or motor impairment
- has trouble with spatial relationships
- does not make eye contact

8. EMOTIONAL DIFFICULTIES

- experiences frequent and unpredictable mood swings or personality changes
- is highly irritable or hard to please
- has high tolerance to pain or is insensitive to danger
- is hard to calm down once excited
- gets frustrated easily
- has temper tantrums and/or angry outbursts
- has low self-esteem
- shows no self-control
- is often anxious
- experiences emotional outbursts
- often gives blank looks or has staring spells
- does not like to be touched
- is destructive or aggressive toward self, others, or property
- is depressed or unhappy

9. BEHAVIOR

- calms down after meals
- has behavior problems or is sleepy two hours after eating sweets
- feels sleepy, droopy, drowsy, or yawns often
- blames others and denies wrongdoing or mistakes
- gives an inconsistent day-to-day performance
- has repetitive behaviors, such as rocking
- is disobedient
- is regularly bored or never satisfied
- is overly assertive or shy and withdrawn
- is accident prone or clumsy
- is unpredictable
- is lethargic

10. POOR PEER RELATIONSHIPS

- hits, bites, or kicks other children
- has difficulty following the rules of games and social interactions
- is rejected or avoided by peers
- avoids group activities; a loner
- teases peers and siblings excessively
- bullies or bosses other children
- has poor leadership ability

11. PHYSICAL SYMPTOMS

- has dark circles or puffiness under the eyes
- has horizontal creases in the lower eyelids
- has chronically swollen glands
- often feels unexplained fatigue
- commonly wets the bed
- has recurring infections such as tonsillitis, colds, sore throats, etc.
- sniffs, clears throat, or wipes nose often
- has respiratory problems
- hears ringing in the ears
- has itchy nose, throat, or skin
- often complains of headaches, stomach or muscle aches

- seems to have a problem hearing, but hearing tests are normal
- is dizzy or nauseous
- feels sick all the time
- is sensitive to certain noises or odors
- has facial tics

12. OTHER CONDITIONS YOUR CHILD MAY HAVE

- hypoglycemia (low blood sugar)
- thyroid problems
- seizures
- asthma
- eczema or other skin conditions

13. EATING HABITS

- craves soft drinks, sweets, or junk food
- covers food with items such as ketchup, mustard, relish
- has trouble facing the day without juice or some particular food
- wants a particular food or drink every day
- has to eat before going to bed in order to sleep well
- is irritable before meals

14. YOUR CHILD HAS KNOWN REACTIONS TO THE FOLLOWING:

- MSG (Monosodium glutamate)
- sugar
- food dyes
- dairy
- fruit
- food preservatives
- wheat
- caffeine
- chocolate
- aspirin
- processed or junk foods
- sugared soft drinks

15. ALLERGIES

- has known allergies to foods, inhalants, or chemicals
- has digestive problems
- reacts to multiple substances that do not seem related (i.e., foods, cats, soaps, pollens)
- complains about odors such as perfumes and cigarette smoke
- symptoms return with each exposure to a particular substance
- has reactions to antibiotics or other drugs
- was on a milk-based infant formula, but did not tolerate it well
- is a picky and finicky eater
- other members of the family are bothered by allergies

16. ENVIRONMENTAL TOXINS

- drinking water contains fluoride
- water pipes in the house contain lead or copper
- pesticides, fungicides, and herbicides are used around the house
- your child's room is over the garage
- your house is newly built

17. HISTORY OF INFECTIONS

- worms or a parasitic infection
- urinary tract infection
- upper respiratory infection
- ear infection
- pneumonia
- sinusitis
- has a history of antibiotic drug use

18. FAMILY INTERACTION PROBLEMS

- frequent family conflicts
- activities and social gatherings are unpleasant
- parents argue over discipline
- meals are frequently unpleasant
- stress is continuous from child's social and academic problems
- parents spend hours with this child, leaving little time for others

- arguments occur between parents and child over responsibilities and chores
- parents, especially the mother, feel frustrated

19. DURING PREGNANCY

- child was active in the womb
- child did not seem to develop normally
- mother used drugs, alcohol, or tobacco
- mother drank milk daily

20. DURING INFANCY

- child did not develop normally
- child acquired babbling or speech then lost it at one time
- child had several milk formula changes

21. DO PARENTS OR GRANDPARENTS HAVE A HISTORY OF THE FOLLOWING?

- allergies
- headaches or migraines
- insomnia
- hay fever
- alcoholism or substance abuse
- diabetes
- asthma
- eczema or other skin conditions
- bad temper
- ADD (with or without hyperactivity)
- manic-depressive illness
- depression

How does your child add up? If you find that several of these phrases describe your child, and you see a certain pattern developing in your child's behavior, your child may have a chronic disturbance such as ADD. This questionnaire cannot give you an exact "yes" or "no" in determining whether or not your child has ADD;

its purpose is to alert you to possible conditions your child may have. In gauging your child's behavior, you have to realize that the range of normal behavior is quite broad. Also, adult expectations for children vary greatly. One person may see a child as restless while another may not. If you did answer "yes" to many of the above questions and are concerned about your child's symptoms, you will need to speak with a health professional about your child. A trained person should be able to provide the proper psychological and medical testing. Your answers to the questions do not, in themselves, indicate emotional health or difficulties. They are simply a point of information for you to use in making decisions about the health and welfare of your child.

Remember that it is important to look for the cause of the behavior, not just treat the symptoms. Once the cause is identified, you can either eliminate negative behavior or treat it. Often the symptoms of hyperactivity and ADD are due to things as simple as what we eat, drink, and breathe. Putting your child on drugs should be your last resort. Always explore the alternatives first.

ADD DIAGNOSTIC CRITERIA OF CHILDREN BY THE AMERICAN PSYCHIATRIC ASSOCIATION

The *Diagnostic and Statistical Manual of Mental Disorders* states, "The essential feature of attention deficit hyperactivity disorder (ADHD) is a persistent pattern of inattention and/or hyperactivity-impulsivity that is more frequent and severe than is typically observed in individuals at a comparable level of development." The following quiz is the only criteria used for diagnosis recognized by the APA. It defines a child as having ADHD if they meet eight or more of the criteria paraphrased here. The list below outlines the criteria. Circle any that apply to your child.

A. (Can be either 1 or 2.)

1. INATTENTION

At least six of the following symptoms of inattention have persisted for at least six months to a degree that is maladaptive and inconsistent with the development level of the child.

a. often fails to give close attention to details or makes careless mistakes in school work or other activities
b. often has difficulty sustaining attention in tasks or play activities
c. often does not seem to listen to what is being said to him or her
d. often does not follow through on instructions and fails to finish school work, chores, or duties in the work place (not due to opposition behavior or failure to understand instructions)
e. often loses things necessary for task or activities (for example, school assignments, pencils, books, tools or toys)
f. is often easily distracted by extraneous stimuli
g. is often forgetful in daily activities
h. often avoids or strongly dislikes tasks such as school work or homework that require sustained mental effort
i. often has difficulties organizing tasks and activities

2. HYPERACTIVITY AND IMPASSIVITY

At least four of the following symptoms of hyperactivity have persisted for at least six months to a degree that is maladaptive and inconsistent with the development level of the child:

a. often fidgets with hands or feet or squirms in seat
b. leaves seat in classroom or in other situations where remaining seated is expected
c. often runs about or climbs excessively in situations where it is inappropriate in adolescents or adults

d. often has difficulty quietly playing or engaging in leisure activities
e. blurts out answers to questions before question is completed
f. often has difficulty waiting in lines or awaiting turn in games or group situations

B. ONSET IS no later than 7 years of age.

C. SYMPTOMS MUST be present in two or more situations (for example, at school, at work, and at home).

D. THE DISTURBANCE causes clinically significant distress or impairment in social, academic, or occupational functioning.

E. DOES NOT occur exclusively during the course of a pervasive developmental disorder, schizophrenia or other psychotic disorder and is not better accounted for by a mood disorder, anxiety disorder, dissociative disorder or personality disorder. In other words, the symptoms are not due to another disorder besides ADD or ADHD.

You can distinguish which type of an ADD disorder your child has by noting which criteria describe your child:

• ADD/hyperactivity disorder is predominately the inattentive type if criterion A(1) is met but not criterion A(2) for the past six months.
• ADD/hyperactivity disorder is predominantly the hyperactive-impulsive type: if criterion A(2) is met but not criterion A(1) for the past six months.
• ADD/hyperactivity disorder is the combined type: if both criteria A(1) and A(2) are met for the past six months.

Chapter 3

WHAT PARENTS
SHOULD KNOW

DON'T ASSUME YOUR CHILD
HAS ADD

D o you believe your child shows signs of ADD? Does your child consistently exhibit undesirable behavior in most settings? The following are steps you should take before going to a doctor to get a prescription for Ritalin or something similar.

- Consult with family, friends and relatives who know the child well. Talk to them about your child's behavior. What types of behavior do they observe your child doing most often?
- Keep notes on your child's behavior.
- Speak to your child's teacher. Teachers often have experience with ADD and can help you reach some conclusions of your own.
- Consult with a holistic health-care provider. He or she will know the medical signs of ADD and will help you make more informed decisions.
- Have your child's eyes checked by an optometrist that specializes

in vision training. It is important to rule out visual problems of any kind.

- Have your child's hearing checked.
- Have your child get a general medical exam. This is very necessary. The medical evaluation needs to include screening for allergies, nutritional deficiencies, heavy metal toxins, and other metabolic disorders. The child also needs a psychological evaluation which includes an assessment of intelligence, achievement, and emotional status.

Parents and teachers should work together and communicate frequently with one another. Since children with ADD have difficulty obeying two different sets of rules, parents and teachers should agree on the same rules and management system. If your child's teachers do not have much knowledge about ADD, you should educate them.

Children with ADD can learn to control some aspects of their behavior. When parents establish and enforce a few rules and maintain a system of rewards, children incorporate such rules into their daily routine. Remember that every child has individual strengths and weaknesses. Once you identify your child's strengths, you can use them to build self-esteem and help provide the confidence needed to tackle difficult situations.

BEHAVIOR MANAGEMENT

Parents of school-age children are likely to complain because the kids are restless, noisy, or difficult to control. Such children are frequently labeled as discipline problems. Their behavior is likely to cause considerable family stress that can in turn make their behavior worse. If causes of negative behavior are not recognized and attended to early, the long-term prognosis will probably be very poor.

Behavior management does not work the same with children who have ADD as it does with children who do not have the disorder. Parenting a child with ADD can be an exhausting and frustrating experience. A simple bit of advice is to not overreact. This can only make the situation worse. Sometimes, parents benefit greatly from a support group.

To decrease a child's inappropriate behavior, parents should use a series of progressively more active responses. First, ignore the behavior. Second, explain to the child the consequences of such behavior. Finally, learn to give commands and directions a child can understand and accomplish. Perhaps the most common complaint from parents is that their child simply doesn't listen. While this is a very frustrating problem, there are ways to increase compliance by applying some of the following strategies.

NON-EFFECTIVE COMMANDS

1. COMMAND OVERLOAD

Giving several commands strung together at a time can result in information overload. For example, "Call the dog, take it for a walk, and then feed it" is just too much information to process. As a result, the child fails to comply.

2. VAGUE COMMANDS

Vague commands do not clearly tell a child what is expected. These include comments such as "be good," "act nice," and "don't make me angry."

3. QUESTION COMMANDS

Parents often ask questions such as "Will you take out the trash?" or "Are you ready to go to bed now?" These types of questions give the child the option of saying "no." If you want to ask this type of question, be prepared for the response you may receive.

4. "LET'S" COMMANDS

Commands such as "Let's clean your room now" or "Let's pick up your toys" give a child the impression that you are going to help them complete the task. Is this your intention?

5. RATIONALE COMMANDS

These are commands followed by a rationale or other verbalization such as, "You need to do your homework, otherwise you will fail your test." These children often do not remember what to do after you give the rationale. Typically children will remember the last statement heard.

EFFECTIVE COMMANDS

Effective commands should be brief and specific. The following are some helpful tips:

- You must first get your child's attention by maintaining eye contact and using a firm tone of voice.
- You should state as briefly as possible what the child is to do.
- Only give one command at a time. Only make a command when you have time to follow through with the appropriate consequences if the child is not compliant.
- Give praise immediately when the child does follow through with the command.
- Give your child about five or ten seconds to comply to a command the first time. A warning or time out may be necessary when the child does not comply with first commands.
- Be prepared with immediate and consistent consequences for noncompliance. Consistency is very important. If your child is not compliant and there are no consequences, or the recourse is inconsistent, the chance of your child's behavior improving is unlikely.
- No child is compliant 100 percent of the time. You should expect to have some noncompliance even after the child's compliance rate improves.

BEHAVIOR CONTROL

Parents can help their children develop more control over their own behavior by having them stop and think before responding impulsively. Place posters with reminders throughout the home. Help your child have a designated area for homework. Color-code clothing drawers. Lay out clothes and other items for school the night before. Establish a daily schedule or routine. Practicing these steps with your child can help them master the strategy. With patience, determination and time, these activities should pay off.

STRUCTURE SITUATIONS

Without consistent structure and clearly defined expectations and limits, children with ADD can become quite confused about expected behaviors. Parents can learn to structure situations in ways that will allow their child to succeed. One mother learned that this included allowing her daughter to have only one or two playmates at a time so that she wouldn't get over stimulated. If your child has trouble completing tasks, you can help by dividing a large task into small steps. As each step is completed, give praise. Children with ADD often require guidance as they structure and prioritize their time. As they grow, they need to be given more responsibility so they can learn from their own decisions.

ORGANIZATION

Another common complaint of parents is that their child frequently exhibits extreme disorganization. This leads to considerable problems with efficient problem-solving. Some tips to help a child learn to solve problems are 1) define the problem, 2) make a plan for solving the problem, 3) implement the plan, and 4) evaluate the plan. Apply this procedure to a variety of problems at home or school, no matter how big or small. Having a messy room or desk, taking too long to do homework or classwork, or losing belongings can all be overcome by recognizing the problem and taking specific steps to overcome it.

SPECIAL TIMES

There is a tendency to label children as hyperactive simply because no one pays the necessary attention to a very active, perceptive, inquisitive, or creative child. Designate ten to fifteen minutes each day as "very special time" to spend with your child. It is important to notice and comment on your child's positive behavior while ignoring, as much as possible, the negative behavior.

WRITTEN AGREEMENTS

Make a written agreement or contract with your child. The child should agree to perform a desired behavior (such as do his homework every night) in return for a desired privilege (such as the right to watch a certain TV show). If the child does not fulfill the contract, revoke the promised privilege. With consistent feedback, a child soon learns to behave in a more acceptable manner. Of course, this procedure may not work as well with young children.

POSITIVE SOCIAL INTERACTIONS

Making and keeping friends is a difficult task for children with ADD. A variety of behavioral problems common to these children get in the way of friendships. They often talk too much, dominate activities, or disrupt games. They may be unable to pay attention when other children talk or they may exhibit inappropriate behavior. Parents need to be concerned about their child's relationship with others. Problems in this area can lead to loneliness, low self-esteem, depression, and an increased risk for anti-social behavior.

As a parent, you can provide opportunities for your child to have positive interactions with others. There are a number of concrete steps you can take:

- Set up a home reward program that focuses on one or two important social behaviors.
- Observe the child in peer interactions to discover good behaviors, as well as poor or absent ones.
- Directly coach, model, and role-play important behaviors.
- Provide praise and rewards when your child shows good behavior.
- Structure activities that are not highly interactive, such as trips to the library or playground.

• Use short breaks from peer interactions when their play becomes disruptive.

STUDY AND HOMEWORK

It may be helpful to have a study area away from distractions. Also, establish a specific time each day for your child to do homework. Do not allow him or her to do homework with the television or radio on, or with other distractions. Another thing you can do to help is when your child has a homework assignment, break it down to its simplest form. Give him only the first part. As he completes each task, move on to the next.

A mother whose kindergarten son had difficulty with complex instructions followed these steps well. When the boy was required to color, cut, and paste, the mother divided up his work. She told him to color a shape first. When he finished that task, she had him cut the shape out. After he finished cutting, she told him it was time to paste, and the assignment was finished with ease. To the mind of a child with ADD all parts of any task have equal importance. The child gets overwhelmed and confused about what has to come first. Parents can easily diminish a child's sense of confusion by allowing breaks and not trying to do everything in one sitting. A reward for any good behavior is beneficial to the child too.

Some other suggestions to help your child keep up with homework are: 1) Note on a calendar long-term assignments and other tasks. 2) Keep the schedule on the refrigerator door, or any other visible place, where it can be a constant reminder. 3) Have the teacher make a checklist of homework to be completed, as well as items to be brought to school the next day. 4) Check the list each evening to make sure your child has completed everything.

REWARDS, PUNISHMENTS AND CONSEQUENCES

Children with ADD require more powerful rewards than other children to motivate them to perform work, follow rules, or behave well. Positive verbal comments are rarely sufficient by themselves. In addition to praise, parents often have to provide physical affection, privileges, special snacks, treats, or points. These things encourage the child to earn something in exchange for desired behaviors. Charts or tokens or stickers can be used to show your child the consequences of good behavior. Points can accumulate for material rewards, such as small toys. Rewards might also include the pleasure of reading, the desire to please one's parents and friends, the pride of mastering a job or new activity, or the fun of having friends over to play. The key is to work on only a few behaviors at a time. As a child's motivation, ability and learning improve, you can give attention to additional behaviors that need correcting.

Don't forget that you need to assist your child in developing personal strengths, not just focusing on weaknesses. Your child already has enough problems—he will only feel worse if you tell him that the task is easy, or that anyone can do it.

Whether or not a child's behavior is good or bad, he needs to know that consequences will be meaningful, immediate, and powerful. Give positive or negative consequences promptly, whenever possible, to establish a strong connection between the behavior and the consequence. Consequences given hours later don't do much good. If you wait until the next day, the behavior may be forgotten entirely. Remember that children with ADD also require behavioral consequences more frequently than other children.

INCENTIVES BEFORE PUNISHMENTS

It is critical to avoid using punishment as the first reaction against unwanted behavior. Remember the rule "positives before negatives" when making behavior changes. Children with ADD typically have a praise deficit and need a lot of positive feedback to foster self-esteem and counter-balance all the negative feedback they get when they misbehave.

When you target an undesirable or negative behavior, you should first redefine the behavior problem—determine what is the desirable or positive alternative. Then watch for that positive behavior, praising and rewarding it when seen. Reward this new behavior for at least a week before you punish the undesired behavior. A mild punishment, when used in conjunction with an incentive program, is a powerful way to create behavior change. This works especially well when only one punishment is being dispensed for every two to three instances of praise and reward.

STRIVE FOR CONSISTENCY

Parents need to be consistent over time. The way you treat a behavior today is how you should treat the same behavior each time it occurs over the next few days and weeks. Inconsistency is one of the greatest contributors to failing in a behavior-change program. Don't give up too soon. For some children it can take months to change.

Your child needs to know that the rules and consequences expected at home also apply, whenever possible, away from home. Anyone who cares for the child should treat him or her in a similar manner. There may be differences in parenting styles between mothers and fathers, but one parent can't punish the child for a certain act of misconduct, while the other one overlooks it entirely.

PLAN FOR PROBLEM SITUATIONS

Children with ADD can be defiant, disruptive, or noncompliant. These behaviors arise not just at home, but frequently in public places such as stores, restaurants, churches, the homes of friends, and school. Parents need to anticipate problems and consider ahead of time how best to deal with their child. A plan needs to be developed and shared with the child beforehand. Parents find it hard to believe that sharing their plan with the child before entering a potential problem setting greatly reduces the odds that behavior problems will arise—but it does! I suggest using the following simple steps to improve the management of children with ADD:

1. Stop just before the potential problem situation and review two or three rules that the child often has trouble following in that situation. Ask the child to repeat these simple rules back. They can be rules such as "stand close" or "don't touch" when entering a department store.

2. Review with the child what rewards he may be able to earn if he obeys the rules and behaves well.
3. Review the punishment that will occur if your child displays the undesirable behavior. Typically, this involve loss of points, the loss of a privilege later in the day, or, if necessary, a time out. Whichever punishment you use, the key to effective management of a child is the immediate consequence when the problem arises.
4. Children with ADD can have "good days" and "bad days." Try to keep your cool and help your child get through the rough periods.
5. Children with attention deficits respond better to consequences, not talk. Parents constantly lecturing the child only make matters worse. When possible, use behavioral consequences instead of lectures or nagging. Children usually behave better in the presence of fathers than mothers. Mothers tend to talk; fathers tend to act.
6. Get individual and family counseling when needed.

KEEP A POSITIVE PERSPECTIVE

When faced with a child who is difficult, parents often lose all perspective. They become enraged, angered, embarrassed, or frustrated when behavioral management does not work. The thing to remember is not to argue with your child about the issue. Arguing is ineffective and may even encourage continued confrontation in the future. At all times, keep in mind that you are the adult. Stay as calm as possible. This may even require disengaging yourself from the encounter for a moment. Walk away as you regain control over your feelings. Remember that children with ADD can't always help behaving the way they do.

PRACTICE FORGIVENESS

Forgiving your child is the most important, but often the most difficult, guideline to practice consistently. After you put your child to bed, take just a moment to review the day. Let go of any anger, resentment, disappointment, or other personally destructive emotions that have surfaced that day due to the child's misconduct or disruptions. Realize that your child may not yet understand why his behavior is bad or may not be able to control it. The child should still be held accountable for misdeeds, but should also be forgiven for them.

Parents should also concentrate on forgiving others who may have misunderstood their child's inappropriate behavior. People often act offensively toward a child with ADD or his parents. Sometims other people simply dismiss the child as lazy, stupid or obnoxious. Such people are often ignorant of the true nature of ADD, typically blaming the parents and family for all of the child's difficulties. This in no way means that parents should continue permitting others to mistreat their children. Education and advocacy for these children are critical so that misunderstandings and mistreatment do not occur again. It is crucial that parents help teach their child's relatives, teachers, and peers about the issues concerning ADD.

The final person with whom you need to practice forgiveness is yourself. Forgive the mistakes you yourself make in the management of your child. Recognize that children with ADD have the capacity to bring out the worst in adults. This frequently results in parents feeling guilty about their interaction with their child. The fact that you make mistakes does not mean that you should not strive to improve your management. You should continue to evaluate how successfully you have approached and managed your child's problem behaviors. Forgiveness means letting go of the self-criticism or guilt that accompany such acts of self-evaluation. Instead of giving way to these feelings, frankly evaluate your performance of the day, identify areas to improve, and make a personal commitment to strive to get it right the next time.

OTHER PARENTING TIPS

- Children with ADD have a difficult time adjusting to changes. Warning children of upcoming changes can lessen the impact.
- Outlining house rules, complete with punishments, is the first step in defining behaviors.

- Time-outs are probably the most widely used form of punishments. These have two benefits: removal of the child from the situation and time for calming down.
- Physical violence against children is extremely discouraged and generally only reinforces negative behaviors.
- Children with ADD function better in a highly structured environment. Remember that consistency is also a form of structure.
- Those with ADD generally do better in the morning. Give them the most demanding work in the morning and let them do something fun later. It's important to realize that symptoms are dependent on the environment; you will not see all the problems in all circumstances.

HELP FOR PARENTS

Inadequate, inconsistent, or ineffective discipline in the home can result in children who have learning problems. Hyperactive children often control the situation in their homes more than the parents do. Parents yield to their child's wishes to avoid confrontation. Children who are disciplined by screaming parents soon stop listening and become uncontrollable. When these children enter school, however, there are limits placed on them. As a result they often manifest overactive behavior as an attempt to control their school environment. Parents must remember that children require discipline. It is difficult at times but there are support groups and other services that will aid in reassuring and strengthening parents of children with ADD. Call 800-632-8188 for the Parental Stress Telephone Counseling Service and 800-348-8437 for Parents Anonymous. See the Resource Guide for more information.

MEDICATION: PROS AND CONS

If your child is taking a drug for ADD, you should request feedback on your child's progress and notify the school of any changes in medication. Drugs are not a cure and should not be used as the only treatment strategy for ADD. You should consult doctors, psychiatrists, and other health-care professionals for advice, but ultimately you must make the final decision about whether or not to drug your child. Remember, there are many effective alternative treatments that do not require drugs.

The short-term benefits of medication often include a decrease in impulsive behavior, hyperactivity, aggressive behavior, and inappropriate social interaction. There may be an increase in concentration, academic productivity, and effort directed toward a goal. However, studies show there are limited long-term benefits of medication on social adjustment, thinking skills, and academic achievements. If you do choose to use drug treatment, you should observe your child for possible side effects.

WORKING TOGETHER

Cooperation and collaboration between the school system, the health practitioner, and the family are keys to developing a comprehensive, successful treatment strategy for a child with ADD. Seek the advice of your school personnel, knowledgeable friends, and national organizations for a referral to a clinician who specializes in the alternative and holistic treatment of ADD.

Chapter 4

A TEACHER'S
INVOLVEMENT

Most teachers today have children in the classroom who are not working up to their ability. Their assignments are unfinished, they put down answers without showing their work, their handwriting and spelling skills are poor, they are restless, talk to others, and they often disrupt class. When the teacher asks the class questions, these children are the ones who shout out the answers without waiting to be called on. They often daydream and seem distracted. Do they have ADD? Are they gifted? Could they be both?

A bright, talented, creative, gifted child could exhibit ADD-like behaviors. Until now, little attention has been given to the similarities and differences between the kids with ADD and gifted kids. This raises the risk of not diagnosing a child correctly. Sometimes, professionals diagnose ADD by simply listening to a parent or a teacher's description of the child's behavior, along with a brief observation of the child. Other times, brief screening questionnaires are used. Children who are fortunate enough to have a thorough physical evaluation have a better chance of being accurately diagnosed. It is always possible that a child may be gifted and still have ADD. Without a thorough professional evaluation, it is difficult to tell.

CONSIDERING THE SITUATION

When a child's behavior is a problem, it is important to examine the exact circumstances of the situation. In the classroom, a gifted child's inability to stay on task may be related to boredom, a mismatched learning style, or other environmental or medical factors. Gifted children often spend from one-fourth to one-half of their regular classroom time waiting for others to catch up. They may be two to four grade levels above their actual grade placement. These children often respond to non-challenging or slow-moving classroom situations by "off-task" behavior, disruptions, or other attempts at self-amusement. This is often the cause for an ADD evaluation. Close examination of the troublesome situation generally reveals other factors that are prompting the behavior problems.

Gifted children and children with ADD may both have high activity levels. Many gifted children require less sleep, but their activity is generally focused and directed. This contrasts with the often aimless behavior of children with ADD. Gifted children can spend long periods of time and much energy focusing on whatever truly interests them. Their specific interests may not coincide with the desires and expectations of teachers or parents. The child who is ADD and hyperactive has a very brief attention span in virtually every situation (except for television or computer games). Gifted children may actively question rules, customs and traditions, and sometimes will create complex rules that they expect others to respect or obey. Some of these children also engage in power struggles. They routinely maintain consistent efforts and high grades in classes when they like the teacher and are intellectually challenged. They may resist some aspects of the work, particularly repetition of tasks perceived as boring. Since difficult behavior and non-adherence to rules and regulations are now accepted as signs of ADD, it may look as if a gifted child has this condition.

One characteristic of ADD that does not have a counterpart in gifted children is variability of task performance. In almost every setting, children with ADD tend to be highly inconsistent in the quality of their performance and the amount of time used to accomplish tasks. Children with ADD typically have problems in virtually all settings, including home and school, even though they can be worse in some settings than in others. Gifted children typically do not exhibit problems in all situations. One teacher may label them ADD while another does not. At school these kids may display the common symptoms of ADD, but not while at scouts or karate lessons.

IDENTIFYING ADD IN YOUR STUDENTS

Many children with ADD are not identified until they enter school and begin to have problems learning class material. The students who should be referred to specialists are those who persistently do not listen and those who give the impression of not knowing what is happening in class. Such children may have difficulty determining what is important and focusing on it. While other children occasionally may become bored with a topic and stop paying attention for a time, children with ADD frequently appear distracted for a long time, regardless of the task assigned. They have difficulty concentrating and often move from one assignment to another without finishing any work. They behave impulsively, without pausing to think about the consequences of their actions. These children seem immature and have behaviors resembling a younger child.

Because the diagnosis of ADD is often based solely on evaluating the child's behavior, teachers must be careful not to single out children who are simply active or overly curious. If you, as a teacher, suspect there is a learning disorder, it is helpful to keep a diary of the child's behavior for documentation, noting how much work the student completes and how often the student leaves his seat. Write down the time of each disturbance and the activity the child is supposed to be doing.

Other factors may cause symptoms similar to those of ADD. They include child abuse, drug use, disorganized home or school environments, and other developmental problems and psychological disorders. Consult with the school's special education staff and counselor to see if they know of other circumstances that explain this child's behavior. Show them your notes. Explain how you attempted to resolve the problems and how the student responded. Contact parents early in the process to describe the problems you are having with their child. They may have concerns of their own and can help explain other factors influencing the behavior.

How to Manage ADD Behavior

Children with ADD respond well to a behavior management system where the teacher gives rewards for good behavior. Concentrate on a few behaviors at a time. Address additional behavior patterns when the child masters the first ones. Students can work toward earning privileges or rewards by gaining points for desired behavior and losing points for undesirable behavior. If you use this system with younger children, you may want to make charts or use stickers to show students the positive results and consequences of their behavior.

You can help children with ADD behave in a disciplined manner in the classroom by establishing a few rules that result in immediate consequences when they are broken. A teacher needs to give immediate feedback so the child understands why he or she is being rewarded or punished. Give the child specific rules, phrased positively, in terms of what the child should do. When you consistently praise and reward the student for good behavior and punish for inappropriate behavior, the child can see that rules are applied fairly.

The teacher should collaborate with a child's parents so that there are not different rules and management systems for school and home. When teachers and parents communicate often, the likelihood that a child will be able to learn effectively is increased. I know of one school that has developed a system which allows parents to give rewards at home for the child's behavior in school. Parents meet with teachers and come to a mutual agreement about targeting specific behaviors. During class, the teacher monitors and evaluates the student. Then, the teacher gives the child feedback and notes on classroom behavior. The child gains or loses privileges at home based on behavior at school.

Teachers can provide a specified time-out location where students can go when they are not in control. This should not be seen as punishment, but a place to go for a few minutes to calm down. Older students need to be taught to sense when they are getting out of control and go to the time-out area on their own. Students who are eleven or older often do better with contracts. If a teacher develops a contract with a student, it must be fair, clear, and positive. Any rewards given based upon the contract should be immediate and systematic.

Students with ADD often need to learn techniques for monitoring and controlling their own attention and behavior. For example, Mark, a boy with ADD, had a teacher who taught him several behavioral alternatives to use when he loses track of what he is supposed to do. He can look for instructions on the blackboard, raise his hand, wait to see if he remembers, or quietly ask another child. The process of finding alternatives to interrupting the teacher has made him more self-sufficient and cooperative. Because he interrupts less, he is beginning to get more praise than reprimands.

Teachers control what goes on in their classroom, and they determine whether or not effective learning occurs. There are many things to consider: the proper learning environment, the giving of instructions and assignments, providing discipline and encouragement. The following list provides suggestions for teachers who have students with ADD.

A PROPER LEARNING ENVIRONMENT

• Carefully select the student's desk placement. Seat them in the front row or near your desk, but include them as part of the class seating. Try not to place children with ADD near air conditioners, high-traffic areas, heaters, doors or windows. Try to find a place that is as allergy-free as possible.

- Surround these students with good role models, preferably students they admire. Encourage peer tutoring and a study buddy. Cooperative learning by the entire class may be another way of encouraging learning, or by dividing the class into cooperative groups.
- Produce a quite study area away from distractions. Let all students have access to this area so the student with ADD will not feel different.
- Reduce the amount of materials present during work time by having the student put away unnecessary items. Have a special place for tools, materials, and books.
- Don't expect students with hyperactivity to sit still for long periods. Plan opportunities for the student to move about or leave the room. You may want to establish active tasks, such as cleaning the blackboard, or leading the class to the lunchroom, as rewards for good behavior.
- Relaxation techniques are important. Non-vocal music playing in the background, stretching or simple yoga exercises, and voluntary "time out" periods work well to enhance a calm environment. The use of headphones with a tape or CD player is a good relaxation idea to use in a classroom.
- Teachers often make their classroom surroundings very stimulating with bright bulletin boards, mobiles, displays, and animals. Make an effort to place these items where they will not cause distraction.
- Encourage parents to set up an appropriate space at home, with set times and routines established for study, parental review of completed homework, and periodic notebook and/or bookbag organization.
- Be creative!

Giving Instructions

- Maintain eye contact during verbal instruction. Do not give instructions while writing on the board.
- Make directions clear and concise. Be consistent with instructions.

- Simplify complex directions. Avoid multiple commands.
- Make sure students comprehend the instructions before beginning the task.
- Students may need both verbal and visual directions. Provide children with a model of what they should be doing.
- Repeat instructions in a calm, positive manner, if needed.
- Help students feel comfortable about seeking assistance. Most children with ADD will not ask for help.
- These children need more help for a longer period of time than the average child.
- Children with ADD do not handle change well, so avoid transitions, physical relocation, changes in schedule, and disruptions whenever possible. You can help the student shift from one task to another by providing clear and consistent transition between activities. It may be helpful to warn them a few minutes before any change in activities.

GIVING ASSIGNMENTS

- Give out only one task at a time. Children with ADD are easily frustrated. Stress, pressure, and fatigue can break down their self-control and lead to poor behavior.
- Monitor frequently while maintaining a supportive attitude.
- Modify assignments as needed. Try to determine specific strengths and weaknesses of each student and apply this knowledge.
- Make sure you are testing knowledge, not attention span.
- Give extra time for certain tasks. Students with ADD often work slowly. Don't penalize them for the extra time.
- Periodically remind student of the assignment.
- Teach techniques for taking notes from both lectures and textbooks. Decrease spelling and copying errors by providing students with duplicated copies of class directions or lecture outlines in advance.
- Incorporate short work periods. Do not assign all work at the beginning of the day since this may be overwhelming. It is also important to give frequent breaks.

- Do not require students to copy questions before answering.
- Give oral tests.
- Give students confidence by starting each assignment with a few questions or activities they can successfully accomplish.
- Vary reading lessons by making use of strategies such as reading together and echo reading (repeating the same phrase several times). Incorporate multi-sensory word activities. These use visual, kinesthetic, auditory, and tactile stimuli to teach sight words.
- Reduce math errors by assigning only a few problems at a time. A large amount of written classroom and homework is usually the most frustrating activity for students with ADD. If the student knows how to do five or ten problems correctly, it isn't necessary to assign twenty or thirty.
- Plan homework carefully. It should be for practice, not instruction. Make sure students can do it independently within a reasonable time.
- Require a daily assignment notebook if necessary. Make sure each student correctly writes down all assignments each day. If a student is not capable of this, the teacher should help. Sign the notebook daily to signify completion of homework assignments.
- Use the notebook for daily communication with parents. A short daily note to parents regarding the student's academic and behavioral functioning is very helpful.
- Send notes to other professionals involved in the child's health care. Professionals may need more extensive communication, but not as often.

PROVIDING SUPERVISION AND DISCIPLINE

- Remain calm, state the infraction of the rule, and avoid debating or arguing with the student.
- Have established consequences for misbehavior before it happens.
- Administer consequences immediately. Praise proper behavior.
- Make sure the discipline fits the "crime," without harshness.
- Avoid ridicule and criticism. Remember, children with ADD have difficulty staying in control.

- Enforce classroom rules consistently. Determine appropriate consequences for all behaviors and follow through in a consistent manner. If students recognize that you sometimes lack consistency in your disciplinary procedures, they will take advantage of this.
- Set realistic behavior goals. These goals may be on a monthly, weekly, daily, or hourly basis. Provide the students with feedback on their progress.
- Have a sense of humor! Humor is a very effective tool to ease tension in the classroom.
- The best way for a teacher to have effective behavior and attention control is to move around the room, rather than remain seated at a desk. Touching a student on the shoulder can redirect the student without calling attention to the situation.

PROVIDING ENCOURAGEMENT

- Reward more than you punish in order to build self-esteem.
- Praise immediately any and all good behavior and performance.
- Change rewards if they are not effective in motivating behavioral change.
- Find ways to encourage the child.
- Teach children to reward themselves. Encourage positive self-talk such as "I did very well on the math assignment today," or "I followed those instructions very well." This encourages children to think positively about themselves.
- Since students with ADD are often rejected by their classmates, successful schools train students with ADD in social skills.

ORGANIZATION SKILLS

- Be highly organized. Material for each day must be ready prior to the beginning of class.
- An organized work area in the classroom is essential. Check the students' desks daily.
- Students with ADD may need more help than their peers in learning strategies to improve their studies and organize their work

more efficiently. Help in these areas may include focusing on listening skills and task structuring.

- Encourage and teach organizational skills. An organized, color-coded notebook can assist the students. It will also help parents when they are checking classwork and homework assignments after school.

MEDICATION IN THE CLASSROOM

Educators generally believe medications are useful for students with ADD and they frequently recommend them to parents. However, most teachers have limited knowledge about the effects of stimulants and receive little education about them. As a teacher, you need to learn as much as you can about ADD, and that includes knowledge about the commonly prescribed drugs for this condition.

Sixty to ninety percent of students with ADD are treated with some form of medication. Due to legal issues, a teacher should never be the one to recommend these drugs. You might suggest that the parents take the child to a doctor for an examination and treatment. Include doctors that treat in a more natural and holistic way, such as Naturopathic physicians. They can also evaluate the child for allergies, nutritional deficiencies, and other metabolic dysfunctions.

If a child's doctor prescribes medication, a teacher should know what type it is, when it should be taken, and what side-effects might be expected to develop. While medication can reduce children's hyperactive behavior temporarily, it does not solve the academic problems experienced by children with ADD. Most studies show that medication has few long-term benefits on academic achievement and social adjustment. Instead, medication is used to make the child more manageable so that the symptoms of ADD are not displayed.

Chapter 5

⌐⌐

THE VALUE OF SELF-ESTEEM

Self-esteem is an attitude that individuals develop and maintain with regard to themselves. It is the approval or disapproval of oneself. Childrens' views and feelings about their abilities and efforts may be different from what others see. Self-perceptions shape self-judgment..

It is important to teach children with ADD that their condition is not "bad." If a child is reasonably intelligent, well loved, and is taught how to use his or her unique traits, great things can happen. For school-age children, the feeling of competence is related to cognitive, physical, and social skills. Children with ADD may ask themselves, "How do I compare academically with my classmates? Do the other students in my class like me?" Their answers will influence their overall feelings regarding "self."

How well can your child complete a task? Can he receive high marks if he works hard at something? Does he know what controls his successes and failures in school? The less he knows the answers to these questions, the less he thinks of himself. A child's perception of his worthiness of love and acceptance from others also influences the way he feels about himself. For mastery of his world and self, he needs positive experiences. A child with ADD is particularly at risk because of noted deficits in the child's emerging sense of self-esteem. This is especially true around the ages of six to eight years of age.

CONSIDER THE FUTURE

Once children with ADD enter school, a major social burden is placed upon them that will last for at least the next twelve years of their lives. The behavior problem becomes a disability to the child, apparent by poor social skills and inadequate school performance. Problems begin to occur with authority. Then there is the embarrassment of taking medication in school. In one case a child would skip lunch because it was the lunch line where the medication was dispensed. Everyone could see who the "stupid kids" were. Often, children do not understand why they need to take medication and other students do not. The ADD label becomes part of the disability.

We now know that ADD symptoms continue for 50 to 60 percent of these children into adulthood. If their self-esteem is allowed to plummet due to the ongoing problems associated with this disorder, this may cause a dangerous spiral of aggression, substance abuse, and conduct disorder.

Starting with your physician, an evaluation needs to be done that does not diagnose just deficits, but also looks for positive individual characteristics. This will lead to a competency-oriented approach to treatment and build self-esteem. The typical approach to the treatment of ADD involves:

- explaining medication management to the child so his self-concept is not compromised.
- educational planning in the school so as not to make the children with ADD seem different.
- making psychological counseling available to enable these children to come to terms with school and family issues.
- encouraging behavior modification to ensure that positive changes in behavior occur.

One of the best ways for improving self-esteem in children with ADD is having them teach certain skills to other students. Perhaps they could tutor or supervise younger children. What does your child do best? Pinpoint a skill and allow him to help others with that skill. It is important to emphasize your child's unique qualities. These could be any type of athletic or academic skills. Coaching an athletic event like soccer can improve self-esteem and social acceptance. Another way to build self-esteem is to have a person who is held in high esteem by the child, such as a principal or a counselor, single the child out for some special assignment. Remember, self-esteem is learned behavior. This cannot be over-emphasized.

There are other ways for your child to build self-esteem. Use individualized activities that are mildly competitive or noncompetitive, such as bowling, walking, swimming, jogging, biking, or karate. Get your child involved in social activities such as scouting, church groups, or other youth organizations that help develop social skills and self-esteem. Allow your child to play with younger children if he or she wants to. Many children with ADD have more in common with younger children than with children their own age. They can still develop valuable social skills.

When a child takes a drug for ADD, parents and teachers tend to applaud the drug for causing the sudden change. This can be dangerous. The child then thinks that they are not responsible for any of the changes. They begin to look to drugs as the answer to solving their problems. The child needs to believe that these changes are actually their own strengths and natural abilities coming out. To help children feel good about themselves, parents and teachers need to praise the child, not the drug.

Chapter 6

DOES YOUR CHILD REALLY HAVE ADD?

At one time or another, most children subject their parents to stress because of their abundant energy or unruly behavior. This is perfectly natural. During certain stages of development, children tend to be inattentive, hyperactive, or impulsive. Preschoolers have incredible energy and run everywhere they go, but this doesn't mean they are abnormally hyperactive. Many teenagers go through a time when they are disorganized and reject authority, but this doesn't mean they will have a lifelong problem controlling their impulses.

Truly hyperactive children, in the pathological sense, have an attention span that is noticeably shorter than other children. Their behavior is more habitual and compulsive than just energetic. They disrupt the classroom by constantly getting out of their seat, talking at inappropriate times, and through general misbehavior. They almost act as if they are possessed. These are not the actions of children that are just badly behaved.

The difficult thing is that many "normal" people exhibit ADD-like behavior at times. Chilren often blurt out things they don't really mean to say, they bounce from one task to another, and what kid hasn't ever been disorganized or forgetful? So how can you tell if the problem is ADD? It is important to consider several critical questions:

• Does your child seem to have any of the previously mentioned traits more than other children you have observed who are about the same age?
• Are the behaviors in question a continuous problem, not just a response to a temporary situation?
• Do the behaviors occur in several settings or only in one specific place (such as the playground or the home)?

Darrell Evans, in his book *Ritalin: A Psychiatric Assault on Our Children,* explains that the problem with diagnosing ADD lies in the psychiatrists' definition of ADD. Of the fourteen symptoms listed in the *Diagnostic and Statistical Manual for Mental Disorders,* many apply to perfectly normal children:

• often fidgets with hands or feet or squirms in the seat
• is easily distracted by extraneous stimuli
• has difficulty playing quietly
• talks excessively
• often acts before thinking
• needs a lot of supervision
• runs about and climbs on things excessively
• has difficulty sticking to a play activity

The ability to learn depends on many factors. Not only do children need to be exposed to instruction and have the opportunity to learn, but they need to be capable of learning. Overall health and emotional comfort are crucial. The mental processes that facilitate learning and the physiological processes that facilitate communication also play a huge role in the learning process. Any sort of irregularity in body systems can result in problems of all kinds. A metabolic imbalance, for instance, could be the result of poor diet, high sugar consumption, excessively active adrenal glands, underactive thyroid function, high copper levels, chemical toxins, enzyme defects, previous infections, and other stresses in life. Disorders of vision, hearing, and speech can also interfere with a child's efforts to learn.

Several other conditions could also be responsible for ADD-like behavior: hypoglycemia, intestinal yeast, parasites, lead poisoning or other heavy metal poisoning. Other possibilities could be exposure to environmental chemicals, fetal drug exposure, birth trauma, or predisposing genetic factors. A large percentage of these children are also allergic or sensitive to foods, additives, and other substances.

Many other things can produce behaviors that look like the supposed symptoms of ADD. Conditions ranging from chronic fear to mild seizures can make a child seem hyperactive, quarrelsome, impulsive, or inattentive. Living with family members who are physically abusive, or addicted to drugs or alcohol, create many similar symptoms. How can a child focus on a math lesson when they feel a sense of danger each day?

What all this really means then is that many children diagnosed with ADD do not actually have the disorder. Symptoms of ADD may really be the symptoms of various other ailments, which doctors group under the umbrella label of ADD. What needs to be realized is that many of these conditions are treatable by themselves. For instance, when a boy displaying the characteristics of ADD is found to have an underactive thyroid and is treated only for that, all the symptoms of his supposed ADD also disappear.

In some children, ADD-like behavior may be their response to a defeating classroom situation. Perhaps a child is just not developmentally ready to learn to read and write. On the other hand, schoolwork may be too easy, leaving the child bored. Disruptive or unresponsive behavior can also be due to anxiety or depression. Sometimes it is just the result of inadequate parenting. Whatever the problem, the children will need a little help to get on track at school, but odds are they don't have ADD.

Is misdiagnosing ADD a huge problem? Dr. Wendy Roberts, Research Coordinator at Toronto's Research Hospital for Sick

Children, did a small pilot study with eleven children diagnosed with ADD. This study revealed that six had true attention problems, but the other five had other learning disabilities or were gifted. She believes that up to 30 percent of children diagnosed with ADD do not have it, but some other problem that interferes with learning and creates behavior problems.

One parent stated that her child did not have the symptoms of ADD defined by the standard tests used by her child's school. Still, the school's physiologist recommended that this child take a sedative drug because of his disruptive behavior in the classroom. When this parent told the child's doctor that he was diagnosed as having ADD by the school, the doctor immediately wrote out a prescription for Ritalin. This was without ever seeing or evaluating the child. Unfortunately, this seems to be a common occurrence.

The following chapters give detailed information on nutritional, dietary, environmental and other factors that produce symptoms or conditions we group under the label of ADD. After reading this book, you will be more aware of what ADD really entails and what you can do to help your child eliminate undesired behaviors, whatever their cause.

Section Two

WHAT YOU EAT— THE NUTRITION AND DIET FACTOR

Chapter 7

⊡

DIET

Diet plays a crucial role in the development and the treatment of ADD. As the saying goes, "We are what we eat." If a child does not eat well, there can be numerous repercussions. Awareness of the food we eat, the use of organic foods, and careful attention to food allergies can all help doctors and parents to change a child's behavior. With a varied and healthful diet, symptons of ADD-like behavior will oftentimes disappear.

THE QUALITY OF FOOD

In the past, the foods we ate were of higher quality. More plants were organically grown and soils were rich in a wide range of important minerals. This was beneficial because plants use minerals just as we do to create necessary chemicals for their own biological function. These chemicals are a part of the food content of plants, and we depend on plants to provide essential chemicals and minerals for us.

In contrast to 100 years ago, today's commercial agriculture artificially creates the appearance of healthy plants by the use of fertilizers, herbicides, fungicides, pesticides, and bactericides. What are generally produced are exhausted crops not healthy enough to survive natural growing without the massive use of artificial and toxic chemicals. Without chemicals these plants could not resist fungus, insects, bacteria, drought, and other manners of stress.

Chemical sprays kill the important soil microbes that help plants absorb minerals into their roots. Commercial fertilizers primarily replace only phosphorus, potassium, and nitrogen. It is difficult for plants to absorb adequate levels of all the important nutrients when they are not available from the soil. Nutrients based upon non-existent minerals can't just magically appear within the plant. Clearly then, when foods are grown organically, they have many more vitamins and minerals, without all the added chemicals.

In the past, meat products were also raised in a more natural and less polluted environment. But our major protein sources today—meat and dairy products—have been altered because of the changes in agriculture. Animals are no longer free-roaming. Their feed contains many pesticides, herbicides, and often antibiotics. With all the publicity about mad cow disease, we now know that it is common practice to add sheep parts to other animals' feed. Food manufacturers can put hormones and other undesirable substances into food without your knowledge. Producers and retailers of grocery stores are not required by law to alert us to the presence of these harmful substances. If you buy processed meat, you are also buying all kinds of additives and dyes.

WHAT SHOULD YOUR CHILD EAT?

Small children eat small amounts of food, so they are dependent on a small amount of food to obtain the nutrients they need. Eating foods that have little nutritional value adversely affects their appetite and decreases nutritional intake. With the elimination of candy, cookies, sugared cereals, soft drinks, food additives and preservatives, many children with ADD make an about-face—they do better in school, improve in physical coordination, and move from being a problem child to a welcome member of the family.

Everyone, adults and children alike, should eat a wide variety of foods. Most people would benefit from eating more fresh fruits and vegetables, seeds, cereals, and whole grains. These foods provide necessary fiber and fluid, high-quality fats, proteins, and the vitamins and minerals necessary for optimum health. The following guidelines outline some suggestions for a healthful, balanced diet.

- Your diet should be high in vegetables, without junk or fast foods. It is a good idea to have a green salad every day.
- Eat moderate levels of protein—it should make up approximately 15 to 20 percent of your calories. Include turkey, fish, or eggs in your diet rather than red meats (if you eat animal products).
- Fat should only make up approximately 20 percent of your calories.
- Complex carbohydrates should make up approximately 60 percent of your calories.
- Substitute organically raised animals and organically grown fruits, grains and vegetables whenever possible.
- Drink plenty of purified water (ideally eight 8-ounce glasses a day). A water purification system in the home is highly desirable to provide pure water for drinking and cooking.
- Remove as many artificial food additives or chemicals as possible from the diet.
- Eliminate foods suspected of containing heavy metals (swordfish, tuna, or canned foods).
- Discontinue sugar, caffeine, and any unnecessary drugs.
- Don't eat the same thing every day.
- Avoid processed foods. The foods that are boxed or canned usually have more additives than those that are frozen. Fresh foods have the least amount of additives, and sometimes none at all. The further removed a food is from its natural form, the more likely it contains additives.

Carbohydrates, fats, proteins, vitamins, and minerals are the basic nutritional building blocks that provide the fuel our bodies need to function and perform. Carbohydrates are our main source of quick energy. Fats, whether solid or liquid, are our primary slow-burning energy sources. For proper brain development, infants need adequate fat in their diet until the age of two. Proteins are the body's chief building materials. Obtaining the right proportion of nutrients is critical to good health. Eating the right number of calories is just as important. Keeping your body healthy is a personal balancing act. The goal is to get the essential nutrients you need, while eating no more calories than your body expends.

The additions of additives, preservatives, pasteurization, homogenization, hormones, steroids, and antibiotics are all good reasons to give up dairy products. It is routine to use Chloramphenicol, a dangerous antibiotic, to treat fevers in cows during their transport. Cattle are also frequently given steroids. All these toxins pass through the milk to you and your child. Unless you have information to the contrary, you need to assume that milk is contaminated and unfit for your child, and you. If you must use cow's milk, consider buying organic milk. It is free of pesticides, antibiotics, and hormones. Health food stores and co-ops usually carry it. Milk also produces excess mucus and some research has shown that milk can leach calcium from bones. Cow's milk causes adverse conditions for many people. Soy and rice milks are excellent alternatives, especially soy milk because it is higher in protein.

Studies in Australia have revealed that high levels of the amino acid tyrosine is present in many hyperactive children. Dietary tyrosine is found in a variety of food products, including yeast extracts, cheese, coffee, citrus fruits, chocolate, and cream. These findings seem to support the idea that a healthful diet can make a difference in a child's level of hyperactivity.

The best kind of diet would consist of 100 percent organically grown, unrefined foods, with absolutely no additives, colorings, preservatives, pesticides, or any other chemical adulterations. This includes avoiding sugar, canned foods, frozen foods, most commercially baked goods, and most restaurant foods. Be absolutely sure of the contents of every item consumed. Even a small amount of the offending chemicals can trigger behavioral problems lasting up to five days. If you only allow one minor slip every five days, and it happens to be the primary irritant, the reaction would be continuous. In this situation, even after a lot of effort and hard work, a child with ADD would still show no improvement.

SHOPPING AT THE AVERAGE SUPERMARKET

Putting together a no-sugar, no-artificial-chemical diet from the average supermarket is not an easy job. The following suggestions will help you find foods with lower chemical contamination.

- Buy lean red meat where the fat has been stripped.
- Buy frozen fish in large pieces or whole fresh fish. Check for preservatives, especially if packaged. Shellfish are better if left in the shell.
- Buy spring-water packed canned tuna, but without MSG. Remember, MSG is called by many names such as "natural flavoring" or "hydrolyzed vegetable protein." (See Chapter 14 for more names.)
- Sardines packed in olive oil or spring water cause less problems than other canned fish.
- Razor clams, shrimp meat, and crab meat vacuum packed in cans from their local city water usually contain chlorine and maybe fluoride. It is best to buy fresh.
- Oysters in glass containers usually have no preservatives.
- Buy nuts in the shell only.
- Sometimes sprayed fresh vegetables are better tolerated if washed and peeled first. Use a food wash to remove as many toxins as possible.
- Eat potatoes peeled; do not bake in skins.

LABEL INFORMATION

The 1990 Nutrition Labeling and Education Act provided the FDA the opportunity to revise the regulations and impose a new structure on current labels. Nearly all labels display their contents and nutritional breakdown. Reference Daily Intakes (RDI) has replaced U.S. Recommended Daily Allowances (RDA). The RDI gives amounts per serving for proteins, carbohydrates, fats, cholesterol, along with some vitamins and minerals. The label focuses on the nutrients that the FDA believes are most important. It does not list all the vitamins and minerals as before.

You should know that the ingredients on a label are listed in descending order based on the quantity used in the product. Sometimes it's hard to be sure what some of the items are. Often there are hidden ingredients, such as sugar. The product may contain several different types of sugars, but each is called something different. Each sugar may be okay in small amounts, but when you add up all the different sugars listed in the product, the total amount is often unacceptable. Terms such as sugar, sucrose, fructose, maltose, lactose, honey, syrup, corn syrup, high-fructose corn syrup, molasses, and fruit juice concentrate are used to describe sweeteners added to foods. If one of these terms appears first or second in the list of ingredients, or if several of them appear, the food is likely to be high in added sugars. A wise shopper reads labels and avoids technical-sounding names that are obviously not natural foods.

It is important to note that a label which advertises "100%" of any substance, such as "100% aloe vera gel," does not mean that the contents of the container are 100 percent aloe vera. It means that the aloe vera used was the entire aloe vera plant, not just the juice or seeds. The product can still contain other substances such as petroleum products, artificial dyes, or preservatives. Such advertising can be very deceiving.

There are various other ways in which labels can be very deceptive. Be aware that labeling on products which says "light" or "lite" does not necessarily mean fewer calories. It can mean that the oil used was lighter in color than the oil normally used. Also be careful to not be fooled by anything labeled "enriched." Manufacturers remove the original nutrients during processing and partly restore them afterwards. Another common practice is to state that a product has no added salt, but the product could already be naturally high in sodium.

In today's market it is also very common to see the word "natural" on a package. Do not be fooled. This does not mean the food is organic or additive-free because many additives are natural substances. It is possible to make an entirely synthetic food from completely natural chemicals. "Natural" may refer to only one ingredient. It could also refer to the processing of the food and not to how it was grown. If you do not know a producer's practices, and if there is no certification label, it is anybody's guess how close the food really comes to being organic.

"Pure" is another misused word. It does not mean a product is additive-free. Unintentional additives such as pesticides and herbicides are sprayed on crops. The hormones and antibiotics given to animals are not on any label. Buy meats that are free of steroids and antibiotics and other toxic chemicals whenever possible. The newest fad is "low fat" items that usually contain large amounts of salt, sugar, MSG, or other taste-producing substances. The irony is that these items may be more harmful than the fat you are trying to avoid.

It is not only national brands that use their labels to deceive the consumer. Analyses of locally made "diet" foods found that soft-serve frozen desserts and muffins often do not live up to their claims. In a New York survey, two types of muffins labeled "fat-free" or "low-fat" contained more than twenty grams fat and about 600 calories. Only one out of ten frozen desserts actually had in it what was stated on the label. The others had at least twice as many calories, sometimes six times as many, as advertised. There was a hefty amount of fat even when the label claimed to be low fat or non-fat. One of the problems was the serving size. A serving of frozen dessert was eight ounces, but the nutritional analyses was based on a four-ounce serving.

Manufacturers know that when specific claims are made on a food-product label, most people believe them and buy the product. Maybe you shouldn't. Make reading labels a regular habit before you toss foods into your shopping cart. Though not all additives must be listed, most are on the package. Compare similar items and choose those that are prepared with the fewest or no additives. When you reduce your consumption of additives, don't overlook sugar and salt. They can also be detrimental to your health.

WHY NOT FAST FOODS?

Fast foods are a nutritional and allergic disaster. They usually contain one or more major food allergens, as well as additives, preservatives, and other chemicals. Sugar is added to poor-quality fast foods to improve appearance and taste. Fast food menus generally do not include fruits, vegetables, and whole grains. Foods such as cheese and shakes are very high in fat. Many sodas contain caffeine, and too much caffeine can cause anxiety, irritability, hyperactivity, muscle twitches, upset stomach, insomnia, rapid heart rate, and nervousness. A steady diet of fast foods and junk snack foods can lead to serious nutritional deficiencies.

WHAT ABOUT ORGANIC FOODS?

"Organic" is the term used to describe the plants grown without artificial fertilizers or pesticides. Farmers who use organic methods grow their crops in a way that enriches rather than depletes the environment. This also includes raising meat without growth hormones, and without antibiotics. Unfortunately, "organic" is being tossed around carelessly by anyone wanting to make some money off this new trend. In 1992, close to 700 new "organic" processed foods and drinks were introduced into the food market.

Consumers have a right to be protected with federal regulations that define and govern the use of the term "organic." Meanwhile, numerous companies are incorporating "organic" into their advertising, implying that their product is somehow better than another. If *organic* or any of the following terms appear on packaged or processed foods there may be good reason not to trust their authenticity: *pesticide-free, local organic, no spray, natural grown with pest management, all natural,* and *minimally processed with no artificial ingredients.* These terms carry no guarantee that they are what we expect when we buy organic foods. In other words, the claim is meaningless.

At present, more than 25 states and many third-party organizations have established certain criteria and procedures for foods before they can carry the organic claim. The Federal Organic Foods Production Act defines "organic" and sets standards for the materials and practices used in the growing and processing of organic foods. The act also creates a national system of farm inspection and certification procedures. Only products labeled "certified organic" or "certified organically grown" by a state agency or a reputable third-party certifier are to be considered truly organic products. These products will carry the certifier's seal of approval or official endorsement.

When you purchase organic foods be sure to look for approval from certifying groups such as the following: California Certified Organic Farmers (CCOF), Farm Verified Organic, Maine Organic Farmers' and Gardeners' Association, Natural Organic Farmers' Association, Ohio Ecological Food and Farm Association, Organic Crop Improvement Association (OCIA), Organic Foods Production Association of North America (OFPANA), Tilth (Oregon and Washington), and the Texas Department of Agriculture Organic Certification Program.

The natural-products industry has gone a step further than the government and considers the term "organic certification of production" to guarantee that not only the ingredients but also the manufacturing processes are certified to be free of contamination from toxic material. Certifying agencies have worked along with manufacturers to develop these standards. If a processed food carries a "certified organic" label, it means that each ingredient and every process qualifies it as organic and chemical-free.

You can usually find a store in your area that specializes in supplying organic foods. A farmer's market or vegetable stand may also supply you with fresh and organically grown foods. These toxin-free foods will improve the nutritional content of your diet.

The best way to replace the important nutrients lost in our current diet is to eat a greater variety of foods, shop for organically grown produce, and cook foods less and at lower temperatures.

Consider adding an organic home garden to your yard. If organic food is not available in your area, there are many mail-order companies listed in the "Resource Guide."

WHY EAT ORGANIC FOODS?

There are various reasons why organic foods are worth the investment. Most importantly, they are better for the consumer than non-organic food. A study done at Rutgers University almost 40 years ago (but buried in obscurity) suggests that organic foods are more healthful than other foods. Organic foods tested in the experiment were more nutritious than non-organic ones. They had a much higher mineral content—calcium was 2.6 times higher in organic snap beans, 3.4 times higher in organic cabbage, 4.4 times higher in organic lettuce, and five times higher in organic tomatoes than their non-organic counterparts. In 1993, another study found that organic produce contained more trace minerals and fewer toxic chemicals than any conventional produce tested.

Another reason organic foods are desireable is that they taste considerably better then non-organic ones. Organic farming starts with nourishing the soil. This leads to more vitamins, minerals, and other nutrients in the plant. The end result is that the food just tastes a whole lot better. You don't have to put sauces or cheese on your food to enhance the taste—good taste is already there.

On the surface, organic foods may appear to be more expensive than conventional foods. What consumers need to realize is that because of the increased nutrition, our bodies will probably need to consume less of an organic food. Even with eating less, the result is added nutrition and better health. Remember too that there are many hidden costs in conventional farming which are paid out by taxpayers: federal subsidies, pesticide regulation and testing, hazardous waste disposal and clean-up, and environmental damage.

FOOD ALLERGIES AND SENSITIVITIES

Most of us grew up believing that dinner was not dinner without a big, healthy glass of milk. The truth is, however, that dairy has more than its share of drawbacks. Many children are allergic to milk. The problem often begins during infancy. A newborn's digestive system is not fully developed and not well-equipped to handle milk protein. When dairy products of any kind, including infant formulas, are introduced too early, an allergy often develops. Many infants and children have rashes, eczema, ear infections, runny noses, asthma, or dark circles under their eyes that begin after milk is introduced into their diets. This premature introduction of dairy may set up a lifelong sensitivity. Wait at least a year to give an infant cow's milk products. If breast milk is not sufficient, goat's milk is a much better alternative.

To avoid food sensitivity in a baby, breast feed completely for at least six months, especially if there is a family history of allergy, hyperactivity, or other behavior problems. It is important that the mother be tested for food allergies or sensitivities. I have found that when a nursing mother has food problems, it often shows up in the baby. Avoid eating large amounts of the same food when pregnant or breast feeding. Delay giving your baby wheat until eight months, citrus fruits and juices until nine months, fish at ten months, cow's milk and eggs at one year, and don't give the child nuts, fruits and vegetables with pips or seeds until he is older than a year. By avoiding these foods until later in your baby's development, food allergies can often be avoided. If you choose to feed your baby table food before age one, stick to homemade pureed vegetables and fruits that are easy to digest. (Allergies will be discussed further in the following chapter.)

LACTOSE INTOLERANCE

Many people confuse milk allergy and lactose intolerance, but they are two different conditions. The enzyme lactase is needed to digest lactose (milk sugar). Most of the world's population, excluding Northern Europeans and isolated groups in Northern India and Africa, are deficient in lactase. Many people of African, Latino, and Mediterranean descent develop gas, bloating, and intestinal cramping after having dairy products. There are now lactase products on the market that can be taken prior to eating dairy products to relieve intestinal discomfort.

SUBSTITUTES FOR WHEAT

Spelt is an excellent replacement for wheat. So is brown rice flour. You can use these flours to create muffins, pancakes, cookies, and cakes. People who don't care for whole wheat products often accept spelt, because it has a milder flavor. Health food stores and co-ops should carry these two flours. Many varieties of grains are available from mail order houses.

HELP YOUR CHILD EAT WELL

Take a serious, long look at your child. Observe her working, playing, and resting. Does she play energetically during the day and sleep well at night? Are her eyes bright and shiny and her skin clear and healthy looking? Apart from the normal challenges associated with developing children, does she seem emotionally stable and pleasant to be around? You will know if something is not right just by observing your child. Some forms of hyperactivity, short attention spans, and mood swings are accepted by many adults as a "phase" that their child will outgrow, or something to be endured or treated with drugs. Don't fall into that trap. The truth is that often these conditions can be corrected by simply eating a healthy diet—fruits, vegetables, beans, and whole grains, as well as a good vitamin and mineral supplement.

Health habits that may profoundly affect your child's entire life are established at a young age. A poor diet not only affects a child now but leads to serious repercussions in the future. The immune system takes a beating from a poor diet. This may explain the reason for the dramatic rise in childhood colds, flu, and serious diseases such as cancer.

Remember that a child is not in control of the food he or she eats. It is up to parents and caregivers to set an example and to offer a wide variety of nutritious foods. Make a commitment to your child that you will never regret. Learn everything you can about eating healthy, and set an example for your child. Encourage him to develop sound eating and health habits that will serve him for years to come. Keep in mind that it is very hard to get children to change their diet without changing the diet of the entire family. Children imitate what they see, so if his dad is having ice cream for desert, your child is not going to accept fruit as his desert. Example is a big part of changing a child's diet.

In the end, there must be diet and lifestyle changes for there to be any permanent cure of ADD. Regulation of diet is a valid concept and a first step in controlling hyperactivity and other health problems. Even the National Institutes of Health said that special diets can help some children. Unfortunately, ADD is treated as if it were a disease. Instead, it may be a case of filling a developing child with toxins, resulting in various symptoms. If you think your child has ADD, get in touch with a naturopathic doctor and seek professional advice on natural therapy.

Chapter 8

⮡

FOOD ALLERGIES

One of the most perplexing problems that can confront a doctor is diagnosing an illness for someone who is suffering from symptoms of unknown origin. Many patients have diseases that are not being correctly diagnosed by conventional medicine. Allergies and sensitivities fall into this category. There is much confusion about the topic of food allergies and sensitivities. The belief of many holistic-minded physicians is that allergies and sensitivities are one of the major sources of illnesses, including ADD, hyperactivity, and other behavior problems.

When people say they have "allergies" they usually mean that they have "sensitivities" to certain foods. A food allergy is a chronic or immediate inappropriate reaction to the ingestion of a food. Broadly speaking, if the immune system is involved in the reaction, it is called an allergic response. If the immune system is not involved, it is called a sensitivity response. This distinction may seem academic, but it is important in order to provide the proper treatment.

It can be difficult to sort out what is actually causing behavior problems. Allergic children are often bothered by their allergies and could appear distracted in class because of their symptoms. If this happens frequently, the teacher wonders why they are not paying attention or finishing their assignment. At home, they might seem fidgety or restless. It can be hard to tell the difference between the symptoms of allergies and the symptoms of ADD.

SYMPTOMS OF ALLERGIES

Symptoms of food allergies and sensitivities can come from virtually every system in the body, including the brain. If your child shows any of the following physical symptoms, they can alert you to the fact that your child is reacting to one or more foods, or to chemicals present in the air, food, and water.

- Gastrointestinal symptoms: canker sores, stomach ulcers, gas, irritable colon, malabsorption, ulcerative colitis, stomach aches, constipation, diarrhea, or celiac disease (an extreme intolerance to a fraction of wheat called gliadin that produces crippling diarrhea and weight loss).
- Genitourinary symptoms: bed-wetting (enuresis), chronic bladder infections (cystitis), kidney disease, fluid retention and bloating.
- Immune symptoms: chronic infections including ear infections and swollen glands under the jaw, armpits, and groin.
- Mental/Emotional symptoms: anxiety, depression, hyperactivity, inability to concentrate, insomnia, irritability, mental confusion, personality changes.
- Musculoskeletal symptoms: bursitis, joint pain, low back pain, and muscle aches and pains.
- Respiratory symptoms: asthma, chronic bronchitis, wheezing, hay fever, and frequent stuffy or runny nose.
- Skin symptoms: acne, eczema (dry or weeping, itchy, thickened, reddened patches of skin usually on the face, wrists and inside elbows and knees), hives and itching.
- Face symptoms: dark circles under the eyes, puffiness under the eyes, horizontal creases in the lower eyelids, pale complexion, and red itchy eyes.
- Other symptoms include irregular heart rate, fainting spells,

fatigue, headaches, hyperglycemia, itchy nose or throat, migraines, sinusitis, and seizures.

If your child experiences any of these symptoms, it is important to determine what causes them. Milk and wheat are two frequent offenders, as are chocolate, peanuts, cane sugar, apples, carrots, tomatoes, eggs, soy, grapes, corn, oranges, red and yellow dye, and preservatives. It is almost impossible to find processed foods that do not contain many of these ingredients. Children and adults suffer because they consume these things several times a day, without a break, and the levels can quickly become toxic.

FOOD AND HISTAMINES

Histamines are chemicals found in foods that often cause allergic reactions. They are responsible for itchiness, skin rashes and increased mucus production. It is a good idea to avoid foods that may contain histamines: sausage, sauerkraut, tuna, wine, preserves, spinach and tomatoes. It might also be necessary to avoid foods that cause an excessive release of histamines from our white blood cells: eggs, milk, shellfish, strawberries, chocolate, bananas, papayas, pineapples, certain nuts, and alcohol. Every person is unique and so are the allergies they suffer. Any treatment for allergies or sensitivities must reflect this principle.

Remember that conventional allergy blood tests such as RAST, Elisa, and the cytotoxic test may not be very revealing. No food or chemical allergy test is perfect, and none cover all types of allergic reactions. Don't be confused if one test shows a specific reaction and other tests do not confirm the allergy. Each test looks for a specific type of reaction and often they do not overlap. Few studies have been performed on the accuracy of allergy tests, but it is known they have their limits. It appears that the incidence of false results may be quite high. When considering any test, it is important to have some idea of the accuracy. There are many articles and books on the subject of food allergies and sensitivities. Do a little research and consult a physician trained in the natural treatment of allergies.

ALLERGY MEDICATIONS

Because allergies are so common, there are many medications available for relief. Asthma medicines and most over-the-counter allergy and cold medicines have some type of decongestant or antihistamine in them. These medications can cause a variety of behavioral symptoms. Different children react in very different ways to antihistamines. Some children become excitable, others get depressed or drowsy. Some become irritable and restless. Most have a noticeably shorter attention span, whether or not there are other symptoms.

Many allergic children have trouble with sleep, either because of their symptoms or their medications. Even if antihistamines make a child drowsy, they still disturb the normal sleep cycles, resulting in daytime drowsiness or irritability. In some cases, allergic children may have enlarged adenoids or swollen membranes in the nose that might cause disturbed sleep patterns.

When a child exhibits ADD-like behavior, it is a good idea to determine if there are any possible allergies that may be causing the behavior. You can't always avoid the offending foods, but here are a few general guidelines that can help to decrease adverse reactions to common foods:

- Eat plenty of foods containing vitamin C, or take a daily supplement. Vitamin C strengthens the cell membranes of the histamine-containing white blood cells.
- Digestive enzymes may be necessary, particularly when eating high-protein meals. Many people suffer from an inflammatory response to undigested protein fragments in the blood stream creating a reaction against the food.
- Take 1-2 tablespoons of essential fatty acids a day. This could be in the form of flax seed oil. Essential fatty acids help decrease inflammatory reactions.
- Vegetables are by far the least allergic foods and high in the vital nutrients that preserve the integrity of tissues. Be moderate with fruit because they are high in simple sugars. One fruit drink a

day is plenty, but always dilute the juice at least 50 percent if you use concentrate. You can even make juice out of your dark, leafy vegetable greens.

Medication is frequently prescribed that suppresses a child's symptoms, but doesn't treat the underlying cause of the problem. A diagnosis of ADD should only be the beginning of your child's journey to health. Testing for allergies or sensitivities is often necessary. A general approach would be to try to eliminate the allergic symptoms by avoiding exposure to the causal food, looking into homeopathic desensitization, or using a less toxic medication that does not cause behavior changes.

If allergies or sensitivities are the underlying cause of your child's learning and behavior problem, sublingual immunotherapy can help. This is a treatment that includes the use of allergen dilutions to block adverse reactions. Sublingual immunotherapy is an effective treatment for food, mold, chemical, and pollen allergies. Children don't mind this type of treatment because they can take each dose by placing drops under the tongue. No injections are necessary.

WHAT ARE BRAIN ALLERGIES?

When an allergic reaction occurs in the brain, swelling and inflammation result. The brain can't produce a rash or sneeze and wheeze, but the allergy is evidenced through changes in thought, mood, and behavior. Brain allergies may cause a wide variety of symptoms that look like mental disorders. Doctors often don't know what to look for so they fail to do the tests that could determine if allergies are causing the symptoms.

The brain is a common allergic target organ and the one most frequently overlooked. In 1971, the first mental illness program was established to detect brain allergies. Doctors found that 90 percent of the patients admitted to institutions had allergies that affected the brain. Any food (especially wheat and dairy), inhalant, or environmental chemical could provoke severe mental symptoms.

One of the brain neurotoxins implicated is tyramine, a natural constituent of some foods, including cheeses, red wine, and chocolate. Additives and incidental food adulterants are other neurotoxins in foods that aggravate ADD symptoms. Ordinary foods can cause some people to act drunk, suffer epileptic seizures, and even attempt suicide. It is rare that a person with a hidden food allergy doesn't have some kind of symptom.

BRAIN ALLERGIES AND ADD

When a child complains at school of headaches, dizziness, or feeling feverish, what does the school nurse do? She takes the child's temperature. If it is normal, the nurse simply returns the child to class and the child is somethimes labeled as a troublemaker. What we have to realize is that a temperature is not the only indication of illness. The most common mental symptoms of brain allergies in children are aggression, irritability, tantrums, mood swings, sleeplessness, depression, anxiety, hyperactivity, learning disorders, the inability to concentrate, and behaving very emotionally. Since the mind and body are connected, the child may also have physical symptoms such as fatigue, muscle weakness and the inability to exercise. A child exhibiting any of these behaviors might not have a temperature, but that doesn't mean he or she has ADD either.

If a child's handwriting, drawing, or behavior shows signs of uncharacteristic deterioration, teachers are likely to call the problem psychological. They label the child ADD and often recommend to the parents that the child be put on one of the current drugs for this condition. What if the inappropriate activity and behavior are not psychiatric, but due to food, chemical, or environmental toxins? School officials need to be more attentive to all complaints and recognize that children's symptoms may be telling us important clues about what is really going on with their health.

Complaints about odors are a common clue to allergies. A brief exposure to a perfume or some other chemical can ruin a child's entire day. The smell signal travels up the olfactory nerve and affects the brain. It can take up to thirty minutes after exposure to a substance before there is a change in the brain's chemistry, but the time it takes to get over the exposure can sometimes be weeks. This is a real problem when there is daily exposure to the offending smell. Sensitive individuals, when exposed to common chemicals, can have brain changes so severe they cause brain injury. Some common toxins that cause reactions are formaldehyde, methyl ketone, ethyl ketone, and acetone. The release of these molecules irritates the brain cells. As people have more and more exposure to chemicals, the risk factors certainly increase.

In the majority of central nervous system allergies, copper imbalance plays a role. High levels of copper are toxic and ultimately result in symptoms associated with brain allergies. The way to handle central nervous system allergies is the same as handling other allergies. Through testing identify and treat any imbalances in the body's chemistry and avoid or be desensitized to the offending substance. Don't just give up if you suspect a child's health problems may be allergy related. Call a naturopathic physician or other holistic-minded health practitioner for more information.

With the identification and removal of specific substances from the diet or environment, a child's mood will improve, emotions will level out, and the mind will clear. The tension, stress, and sleeplessness will simply disappear. Any allergy sufferer can return to normal. The next time your child's behavior becomes undesirable, look for the solution as close as your grocery shopping cart, or the odors around you.

EASY SELF-TESTING

When using allergy tests, the particular test you use can make all the difference in the results you get. The following are the types of self-tests you might use to detect food, chemical, and airborne allergies and sensitivities. Each method has its limitations.

• ELIMINATION-THEN-CHALLENGE DIET

The elimination-then-challenge diet is one way of removing dietary stress and allowing the body to heal. This test involves completely removing a suspected food, or several foods, from the diet and closely observing if symptoms improve. Later, the food is reintroduced (the challenge diet) to see if the original symptoms reappear. In this way you can determine what foods cause allergies. This is one of the most simple and economical methods.

Elimination-then-challenge type of testing is not always successful, however, because most people have problems with several unsuspected foods. The test is also very subjective, time-consuming, and only useful to people who have noticeable symptoms. (See chapter 16 for more information.)

• JAR TEST

This is usually a good test for inhalant or brain allergies caused by perfumes, cleaning products, fabric, carpet, flowers, house dust, animal dander, or mold. Put the allergen suspected of causing the problem in a jar. Leave the jar in the sun for a short time. Take off the lid and smell the substance. Note any reaction that may occur. It can take thirty minutes after exposure before there are changes in the brain and symptoms begin. It can take minutes, hours, or days before the symptoms disappear. This test will easily verify any suspected inhalant allergies.

• PULSE TEST

This test is based on the reactions of two closely spaced feedings after a period of avoidance. The foods to test are those a child eats at least twice a week. You will need to ensure that your child absolutely avoids any form of the food for at least four days before testing, but not more than ten days. When omitting many of the basic foods such as corn, wheat, yeast, egg, milk, beef and pork, be aware that many commercially prepared products contain these ingredients. During a period of food avoidance, it is common to have withdrawal symptoms that usually clear by the end of the third day.

Before starting this test, write down all the symptoms your child is presently experiencing, such as stuffy nose, cough, throat clearing, sneezing, tiredness, fatigue, headache, itching any place, nausea, vomiting, diarrhea, abdominal cramps, urinary frequency and behavior problems. The types of symptoms will vary according to the individual's problem. During the middle of the day on the fifth or sixth day of avoidance set aside two hours for performing the test. During this two-hour period avoid other activities.

Take and record your child's pulse for one full minute before eating. Place two fingers over the artery just inside the wrist of the opposite hand, but don't use your thumb because it has a pulse of its own. Then have your child eat an ordinary serving of one specific food at the designated time, within a five-minute period. Make sure he eats only the test food. Do not add anything to the food, not even salt. If you need to cook the food, then use glass or stainless steel pans and utensils. Use only distilled water during cooking.

Now, take and record the pulse for one full minute after finishing eating, and again twenty, forty, and sixty minutes following the meal. If the pulse goes above eighty-four beats per minute, or if there is a variation of more than ten beats per minute, this would suggest an offending food. Observe any symptoms during these intervals and write them down as they occur.

A pulse increase without symptoms indicates a probable sensitivity. If definite symptoms do occur, the test is positive for that particular food. Observe any symptoms that occur over the next 30 minutes. If you do not observe any symptoms, include the test food with the next meal. Watch for delayed symptoms during the night or the next day.

The main disadvantage of this test is that only one body function is being considered, a change in heartbeat. One-third of allergy-prone people will have an increase in pulse rate while another one-third will experience a decrease. The other third will experience no change. This response may differ at various times depending on what foods are consumed. This test is valid only if there is a definite, consistent change in the pulse rate. Another confusing factor is that you can have a reaction to a food as long as three days after eating it. The pulse test is not 100 percent reliable for a diagnosis of an allergy or sensitivity, but it is a good place to start. It gives you one possible way to determine a food reaction.

If any food test is positive and the symptoms are especially uncomfortable, it is advisable to take a natural laxative to clear the intestinal system of the offending food. You may want to contact your physician before starting any self-test so you will have something on hand to neutralize any possible food reaction.

MORE PROOF

Children with behavior disorders usually experience significant improvement with a low allergen diet. Many even achieve a normal range of behavior. World-renowned retired pediatrician and author, Lendon Smith, M.D., reports that 80 percent of children get better just by changing their diet and taking vitamins. He is a pioneer in the field of food sensitivities and child behavior. Dr. Smith believes that food sensitivity is the key factor for many of the children with ADD. He says that these same children are also more susceptible to blood sugar fluctuations. Children with food sensitivities and blood sugar problems are the "Jekyll and Hyde" type kids who experience drastic mood swings. When you eliminate the offending food(s), supplement the child's diet, and stabilize the blood sugar, the child will usually get better.

Dr. William Crook, M.D., a pediatrician from Tennessee, has used a natural approach to hyperactivity for twenty-five years. In a study reported in the *Journal of Learning Disabilities* (May 1980), he published the observations of parents of 182 hyperactive children. A majority of them said that their child's hyperactivity was definitely related to specific foods. Sugar was the worst offender, followed by food additives, and then common foods such as milk, corn, wheat, and eggs. Dr. Crook says that 94 percent of the hyperactive children he has seen are allergic or sensitive to foods or food colors of some sort. With a healthy, organic diet there is a good chance that a child's behavior problems can be controlled without the use of drugs.

Chapter 9

⑬

BIOCHEMICAL
FACTORS

Conventional medicine pays little attention to nutrition as a cause of ADD. Many researchers, as well as psychologists and psychiatrists, virtually ignore the link between behavior and body chemistry. The fact is that behavior and learning disorders are often a result of nutritional imbalances. Dr. Paul C. Eck of Applied Nutrition and Bioenergetics in Phoenix, Arizona, has worked with hair trace-mineral analysis for the past twelve years and has reviewed over 125,000 mineral profiles. He has identified several clear biochemical patterns associated with hyperactive behavior and by correcting these biochemical imbalances has reduced negative behavior.

It is known that a dysfunctional body chemistry may not be the only cause of hyperactivity or behavior problems, but in many cases it may be the most important factor. Any chemical imbalance can add to a child's total stress threshold. Reducing this threshold to a certain level eliminates the symptoms of ADD, or at least certainly reduces them. Biochemical factors are worth looking at because they can be measured and monitored objectively. Correction is possible through diet changes and nutritional supplements.

Five major types of biochemical imbalances are thought to be the principal causes of hyperactivity, learning disability, and other related disorders. Dr. Eck's hair trace-mineral tests can identify the underlying cause(s) which might contribute to ADD:

- Mineral deficiencies/imbalances
- Copper imbalance
- Overactivity of the adrenal glands
- Exhaustion of the adrenal glands
- Elevated toxic metals

MINERAL IMBALANCES

SEDATIVE MINERALS

A hair trace-mineral test often discloses an excessively fast oxidation rate along with low levels of the sedative minerals: calcium, magnesium, and zinc. Many children have low calcium levels despite drinking plenty of milk. Excessive salt intake can lower tissue calcium, magnesium, and zinc levels and contribute to an increase in activity. Behavior that could be mistaken for ADD can be normalized with supplements of sedative minerals

SODIUM-POTASSIUM IMBALANCE

If the mineral levels of sodium and potassium are not in the proper ratio, a child can have increased nervous excitability and irritability. The child may even be aggressive and violent, especially when tired or feeling threatened. Sleeping may also be a problem. Parents and teachers who try to discipline the child will wear themselves out quickly. Quick solutions often will not reveal the real cause of the behavior problem.

Ritalin, a stimulant drug, has a sedating action when given to hyperactive children. Ritalin appears to raise the activity of the adrenal glands, which raises the sodium level, which in turn raises the blood pressure. This tends to temporarily normalize the sodium/potassium imbalance or temporarily improve adrenal gland activity. The child then has more energy to cope with stress and is able to calm down.

PHOSPHORUS LEVELS

High levels of phosphorus and very low levels of calcium and magnesium usually indicate a potential for hyperactivity and seizures. Phosphorus levels can be determined through a hair trace-mineral analysis. If your child's levels are elevated, then a low phosphate diet may be indicated. Carbonated drinks are high in phosphorus, as well as red meat and fat.

IRON DEFICIENCY

In 1992, the *American Journal of Diseases in Children* cited a study indicating that iron deficiency is the world's most prevalent nutritional disorder. This deficiency is associated with a markedly decreased attention span, decreased persistence, and decreased voluntary activity. Research shows that teen-age females experience significant improvement in overcoming fatigue, their ability to concentrate in school, and controlling mood. An iron deficiency (which can cause anemia) is important to treat because an iron-deficient child is more likely to absorb toxic levels of lead.

ZINC DEFICIENCY

A low zinc level is associated with hyperactive behavior. Zinc is a sedative mineral that prevents the nervous system from over-responding to stress. A zinc deficiency is common today because refined foods are low in zinc, stress depletes zinc reservoirs, and the soil is deficient in zinc in thirty-two states. Also, many children are born to mothers that are already zinc deficient.

COPPER IMBALANCE

A copper deficiency frequently develops after prolonged or recurring infections. This leads to a vicious cycle of more infections and increased hyperactivity. If the cycle continues, ADD could be mistakenly diagnosed. Certain antibiotics, such as penicillin, decrease copper levels. Children are normally born with a high level of tissue copper. This high level at birth serves to protect against the excessive level of stress that occurs at that time, but it is not healthy to maintain that level later on.

A copper imbalance may or may not be detectable on a serum blood test. Using a hair trace-mineral analysis as a testing procedure clearly defines if the copper level is normal or toxic. Correction of these minerals imbalances often causes dramatic improvement in concentration, behavior, and social interaction.

In some hyperactive and learning-disabled children, copper can be present in toxic amounts in body tissues, and at the same time be unavailable for use by the body. This condition is known as bio-unavailability. It seems that copper cannot be released in normal amounts from liver and brain storage when the adrenal glands are not working properly.

OVERACTIVITY OF ADRENAL GLANDS

Some children seem normal at home, but have trouble in school, especially when placed in a stressful situation. They are more reactive to stress and have difficulty remaining calm. The sedative minerals are often an important part of the nutritional correction of ADD and hyperactivity disorders. These minerals help to slow overactive adrenal and thyroid glands, and reduce the "fight-or-flight" reaction.

Some children have overly active adrenal glands because of genetic, biochemical, or neurological defects. More commonly, it is due to an impaired biochemistry from the parents, especially the mother, who can pass it to her child during pregnancy. If a mother was over-stressed, had a poor diet, or suffered from copper or other toxic metal poisoning during pregnancy, it could contribute to her child's biochemical imbalance.

Chronic infections, such as earaches, colds, sore throats, and allergies also increase the activity of the adrenal glands. Research indicates that children with low tissue copper levels, in addition to low calcium, magnesium, and zinc levels, are more prone to infections. The link between a child with chronic infections, low mineral levels, and hyperactivity becomes apparent.

Along with low copper levels, a deficiency of manganese can cause adrenal exhaustion. Manganese, iron and copper are also required for energy production and optimal adrenal gland activity. A child may eat foods adequate in minerals, but children with ADD often need three or more times the recommended amount of certain nutrients in order to balance their body chemistry.

LOW SUGAR RESERVES

As the child's body continues to be hyperactive, it uses up the glycogen (sugar) reserves in the liver, resulting in a sudden drop of blood sugar. This produces anxiety, nervousness, irritability, fatigue, and mental confusion. Erratic behavior and mood swings may also occur. Children already have a fast metabolic rate. If they also tend to be hypoglycemic, they have little reserve glycogen. They need to learn to eat right or their blood sugar is going to drop and undesirable symptoms will occur. A low blood sugar can also occur in those with underactive adrenal and thyroid glands. This usually results in a craving for sweets and can directly influence behavior.

Cognitive disturbance in children may result from inadequate supplies of minerals such as chromium. Chromium is required for regulating blood sugar levels. Many hyperactive children are sugar and carbohydrate intolerant which leads to severe mood swings.

EXHAUSTION OF
ADRENAL GLANDS

LOW THYROID FUNCTION

Hypothyroidism in childhood severely limits development of the brain and may be an important component of hyperactivity and ADD. Body cells need the thyroid hormone in order to produce enough energy to become quietly relaxed. For many years, physicians have known about the quieting effects of thyroid hormone and have prescribed it for hyperactive children. Physicians using the Barnes method of diagnosing a low functioning thyroid (taking the basal body temperature) find that at least twenty percent of their patients have subclinical hypothyroidism. It seems probable that a subtle form of thyroid hormone resistance could exist in some of these children.

LOW ADRENALINE

According to researchers Mefford and Potter, most of the hyperactive children receiving drug therapy in the U.S. are suffering from low adrenaline (*Medical Hypotheses* 29:33-42). They have found that low adrenaline in children creates the same hyperactive symptoms of ADD—difficulty focusing attention, restlessness, and difficulty understanding and solving problems. As a result these children cannot filter out all the incoming stimuli. This inability results in excessive activity on the part of the brain that regulates aspects of attention and sleep. If brain activity becomes extreme, adrenaline can help calm a child. The use of Ritalin and similar drugs relaxes these low-adrenaline children by helping to produce adrenaline, or mimicking its effects. In people with normal adrenaline amounts, however, amphetamine drugs like Ritalin can raise levels too high and create anxiety.

Dr. Timothy Jones of Yale University did a study on how sugar affects adrenalin production. A group of adults and children were given the sugar equivalent of two 12-ounce colas. The blood glucose levels recorded similar highs and lows, but the adrenaline level of the children was twice as high as those of the adults. More of the children felt weak and shaky. As a result of this study, Dr. Jones advises that children not be given sweets on an empty stomach. He also suggests that an increase in adrenaline could be linked to the hyperactivity some children display after eating sweets.

THE REMEDY FOR BIOCHEMICAL IMBALANCE

In a school for "impossible" children, student's behavior improved under a treatment that incorporated food and vitamin/mineral therapy. Teachers were startled to see the difference that nutrition played in health and behavior. This treatment program was based on the book *The Orthomolecular Approach to the Treatment of Children with Behavior Disorders and Learning Disabilities*, published in 1977 by Dr. Allan Cott, a New York psychiatrist. He examined the biological and chemical basis for learning disabilities and their treatment. The study showed that the correction of even mild nutritional deficiencies had a substantial influence on learning and behavior.

Modern diets are deficient in trace minerals and frequently deficient in vitamins as well. Any nutrient deficiency can result in a stress on the body. A vitamin B-12 deficiency may cause severe psychiatric symptoms that can vary in severity from a mild mood disorder to paranoid behavior. There has been credible information available for decades that nutritional deficiency can result in impaired brain function. Some studies have shown that the presence of excessive amounts of individual B vitamins may keep other vitamins from working properly. Megadoses of vitamin B-6 may be capable of inducing a significant folic acid deficiency. Don't give your children megadoses of vitamins or minerals without guidance from a trained nutritional health professional.

An article in the *Journal of Advancement in Medicine* discusses the relationship between nutrition and criminal behavior. The authors found evidence that in young, first-time criminal offenders there is an abnormal central nervous system biochemistry resulting in basic behavioral distortions. The exciting thing is that after nutritional and dietary counseling and treatment, the symptoms disappeared. Obviously, there is a need to look for any malnutrition in the presence of unexplained violence, conduct disorders, poor academic performance, and low nonverbal intelligence.

The *Journal of Applied Nutrition* (1991) reviewed some similar studies done on nutrition and behavior performed at California State University over the last decade. It was found that nutrient-dense diets resulted in significantly improved conduct, intelligence and/or academic performance. Children placed on vitamin and mineral supplements exhibited significantly less violent/antisocial behavior, higher gains in nonverbal intelligence, and higher academic achievements than children on placebos.

One of the studies also found that children who took 100 percent of the RDA did better on IQ tests than those receiving 200 percent or 50 percent of the recommended formula. It seems that taking the higher amounts of minerals inhibited vitamin absorption. A key finding in these studies was that while there is definite improvement with vitamin supplementation, taking more is not always better. Too much of a good thing can cause symptoms like a low-grade fever, fatigue, loose stools, vomiting, rash, and hair falling out. A one-year-old boy had these symptoms for six weeks because his mother had given him megadoses of vitamins, especially vitamin A, He improved dramatically when the vitamin supplements were stopped, without any other intervention.

Please be aware that vitamin and mineral deficiencies are especially likely during growth spurts. These are the times when a child's nutrient needs are highest. There is even a greater danger if your child is also taking the common ADD drugs that suppress appetite. Make every attempt to encourage your child to eat a variety of fresh and wholesome foods, such as fresh fruits and vegetables, lean meats, and cooked beans and peas.

Avoid nutrient-poor foods, commercial snack foods, and sugary foods. Do not drink water treated with a water softener. It removes vital trace minerals such as magnesium and calcium. Buy a water filter that does not remove the minerals, only contaminants. If it removes minerals, you need to replace them with supplements. Some water filters also harbor bacteria. Distilled water is not always a good choice either, because it has the minerals removed. Have your child take a multiple vitamin-mineral preparation containing approximately 100 percent of the fat-soluble and water-soluble vitamins, calcium, magnesium, and trace minerals. Of course, it is important to discuss any treatment with a physician who has training in nutritional therapy.

Chapter 10

⎍

HYPOGLYCEMIA
AND ADD

Hypoglycemia is a deficiency of glucose (sugar) in the blood. This condition is responsible for a great deal of suffering that most of its victims do not understand. It is also known as "functional hypoglycemia" or "reactive hypoglycemia." Absolute proof of hypoglycemia will not always be revealed with a glucose tolerance test. If the symptoms are present, a trial diet will usually help. Fortunately, this problem is curable, or controllable in most cases, with proper dietary management, nutritional supplements, and stress management.

All cases of behavioral and emotional problems should be evaluated for blood sugar abnormalities, food allergies and sensitivities, or endocrine imbalances. New medical research supports the view that the effects of hypoglycemia may be behind a significant proportion of mental and emotional disorders, including hyperactivity, antisocial behavior, criminal personalities, drug addiction, and allergies. In a large-scale study, 200 hyperactive children had low blood sugar often enough that it started or aggravated typical hyperactive behavior. Many of these children also had allergies to common foods. These were usually those foods that they favor and eat whenever possible. This sets off abnormal behaviors, many of which are the same ones found under the diagnosis of ADD. In another study with 265 hyperactive children, it was found that glucose tolerance tests were abnormal in 76 percent. This suggests that abnormal glucose metabolism may be a factor in the cause of hyperactivity.

WHAT ARE THE SYMPTOMS?

Low blood sugar creates a wide array of psychological symptoms including behavioral changes. The most common food-mood connection includes symptoms such as the inability to concentrate, mood swings, anxiety, depression, and being more emotional than usual. Other symptoms include asthma, fatigue, headache, hyperactivity, nervousness, insomnia, irritability, restlessness, poor memory, and indecisiveness. A child exhibiting this behavior could easily be assumed to have ADD when really the child is the victim of a bad diet. The supposed ADD symptoms are simply caused by unstable blood sugar levels.

WHAT IS BLOOD SUGAR?

The brain and other body tissues must have a steady supply of glucose (energy) to maintain health. The bloodstream carries this fuel source to all parts of the body. There always must be a certain amount of glucose in the blood to guarantee that the entire body gets its adequate share. If the level of glucose in the blood drops below normal, low blood sugar results.

While all foods contain energy, different foods may affect the blood sugar in different ways. Simple carbohydrates, or sugars, absorb very quickly from the intestines into the bloodstream. If you continue to eat these sugar-type foods, the body overreacts and much more insulin is produced than the body needs. This overflow results in a large amount of blood sugar being absorbed in a short amount of time. The blood sugar then drops dangerously low. Mental, emotional and physical changes may begin as the energy level decreases. Depression, anxiety, fatigue, or many other symptoms can occur. What, then, does a child with hypoglycemia do? Just what any of us might do—reach for sugar.

This type of sugar craving begins a vicious cycle. The child eats the candy bar or soda and feels revitalized from the quick "up" that the suagr gives. Soon, the sugar load overstimulates the pancreas and a burst of insulin comes pouring forth. Promptly, the blood sugar level drops lower than before. What does the child do next? There is only one recourse—that is to eat more sugar. This, however, is only a short-term solution that ultimately repeats the problem it is meant to solve.

WHAT CAUSES HYPOGLYCEMIA?

The two most significant factors contributing to hypoglycemia are diet and emotional stress. The average child's diet is almost a prescription for hypoglycemia. Common foods like white bread, sugar, and soda pop contain refined carbohydrates which absorb very rapidly into the bloodstream since they require little digestion. Most people fail to recognize that excess table sugar is not the only refined carbohydrate that may lead to hypoglycemia. Excess honey, fruit, fruit juice, dried fruit, and sometimes vegetable juice will cause a rapid rise in blood glucose levels.

Stress also affects blood sugar levels. First, stress depletes the B-vitamins and vitamin C, both necessary for proper adrenal function. Yet it is the adrenal glands that recognize stress as an emergency. Stress requires adrenal glands to work overtime, and at the same time strips them of what they need to function.

Another blow to the adrenal system is that refined foods are also stripped of needed vitamins. The empty calories we consume do nothing to help our body. Yet another problem is caused when we drink caffeine. Caffeine stimulates the adrenal glands to mobilize the body's energy reserves in both the liver and muscles. This in effect nullifies the body's backup mechanism to keep the blood glucose level balanced and further abuses the adrenal glands.

How do we stop this ugly cycle? How can we maintain our blood sugar levels without abusing our body? By using one particular food group that will positively influence our moods, our ability to think,

and our energy levels—complex carbohydrates. Complex carbohydrates are more efficiently used and more readily available as a source
of energy than either fats or proteins. They digest easily and enter
the bloodstream quickly.

Simple carbohydrates are foods that breakdown to glucose very
easily and enter the bloodstream too fast, causing rapid elevation in
the blood sugar, followed by a quick drop in glucose levels. This
drop will affect a number of brain-related functions and can result
in slow reflexes, an inability to concentrate, fatigue, hunger, and a
light-headed sensation. Refined carbohydrates and sugars are
usually void of the vitamins, minerals, fiber, and other micro-nutri-
ents required for the transformation of glucose into energy. When
simple carbohydrates are the main part of the diet, hypoglycemia is
usually present.

Because we want to avoid hypoglycemia, the bulk of our diet
should be in the form of complex carbohydrates. Found in most
vegetables and whole grains, they replenish glucose at regular intervals, keeping the body's energy constant. Complex carbohydrates
and unrefined starches from whole foods can provide the necessary
nutrition that the body needs to maintain a stable blood sugar.
Without health-giving nutrients, the body must use its valuable
reserves and easily becomes depleted.

CURING HYPOGLYCEMIA

If all conditions were as easy to treat as hypoglycemia, the world
would be an Eden of wellness. This is not an over-simplification. A
change in diet can mean a change in behavior, a change that means
the elimination of ADD-like behavior. The main things required of a
sufferer of low blood sugar are: first, to stop eating sugar, caffeine,
refined carbohydrates and second, to learn how to have a healthy diet.

TREATING HYPOGLYCEMIA WITH DIET

1. All sugar intake must stop. Most of the children affected with
hypoglycemia have a poor diet history. They usually have a breakfast

of a sugared grain cereal with milk, lunches and suppers of fast foods, and snacks filled with sugar. They eat foods full of preservatives, dyes, and other chemicals and pesticides. The common drinks are usually milk, some sugar-laden soda, or a sugared fruit drink. This type of diet is more than likely deficient in fresh vegetables, fruits, and adequate water.

It is important to note that some people with hypoglycemia do not function well on fruits. If you are in this group it is best to avoid fruit, at least initially, in your diet management program. Hypoglycemics should also avoid all fruit juices, dried fruits, and even some vegetable juices. These are concentrated forms of sugar even in their natural states and evoke low blood sugar reactions minutes to hours after eating. It is best to eat whole fruits because they contain more fiber and less concentrated sugar. Grains and vegetables also provide time-released glucose.

2. The diet to cure hypoglycemia stresses adequate protein and complex carbohydrates. Protein in this case includes moderate amounts of fish, lamb, turkey, and chicken. It is best to avoid the more dubious varieties of meat like hot dogs, chain-store hamburgers, and high-nitrate lunch meats. Other good sources of protein and complex carbohydrates include eggs, green leafy vegetables, dried peas and beans, brewer's yeast, whole grain cereals, soybeans, lentils, bean curd (tofu), sunflower seeds, pumpkin seeds, kefir, peanuts, almonds, cashews, soy flour, wheat germ, fresh fruit, and vegetables. With few exceptions, the high-protein diets advocated in the past for hypoglycemia may make the condition worse.

The ideal diet for most people will be about two-thirds complex carbohydrates. But because of biochemical individuality, some individuals do not do well on a diet rich in carbohydrates. These are people with fast metabolisms. They burn their foods too fast and seem to do better when additional protein is added to their diet. Also, some people are carbohydrate-sensitive and do not thrive at all on carbohydrates.

3. The ideal approach to overcoming hypoglycemia is to eat several small meals a day rather than three large ones. It is also important to eat only when hungry, not according to the clock, and to not skip meals. Five or six somewhat lean feedings are best, with plenty of fresh food. Try a small breakfast, a good mid-morning snack, a light lunch, a mid-afternoon snack, dinner, and a snack before bed. The point of eating a little food at frequent intervals is to maintain a certain amount of naturally-derived sugar in the bloodstream to maintain proper blood sugar levels.

4. Children need dietary fats and oils to grow. Many vital body tissues require fatty acids to function properly. Children who are fast oxidizers need fats to calm them down, provide steady energy, and avoid the energy roller coaster of hypoglycemia. Deprived of healthy foods, children often crave and eat more sugar, leading to sugar addiction. Feed your children regular meals and teach them good eating habits.

5. The following are guidelines you can employ in managing your child's diet (as well as your own):

- Eat enough to prevent hunger, but do not persist until stuffed.
- Eat three small meals daily and have frequent snacks instead of gorging on a few large meals.
- Eat on a regular schedule; don't skip meals.
- Eat quality proteins and complex carbohydrates. Don't eat more than two pieces of bread daily.
- Eat only a moderate amount of fat. Include adequate EFAs.
- Avoid foods high in refined sugars and artificial sweeteners.
- Eat fresh vegetables, steamed or raw, as well as two servings of fresh fruits daily. Eat fruit alone. Avoid fruits packed in syrup.
- Avoid certain foods if your child exhibits even a touch of hypoglycemia. These foods are refined white flour, dried fruits, soft drinks, caffeine, citrus drinks and fruits, black tea, and salt. Also, beware of foods containing cocoa with a sugar base.

• It is good for your child to eat heartily and often when suffering from hypoglycemia. But remember that overeating causes the blood sugar to drop. Just use common sense.

HOW TO DEAL WITH SUGAR CRAVINGS

Foods such as walnuts, bananas, and fresh pineapple may help reduce sugar cravings. Usually after a week or so with no sugar in the diet and the stabilization of the blood sugar, the craving for sugar goes away. Pantothenic acid (100 milligrams) may be chewed whenever the craving for sugar becomes strong. Mineral supplements high in magnesium and trace minerals are helpful to decrease sugar craving. Bile salts can reduce craving for sweets in some people. The cell salts useful for sugar cravings are silica, magnesium phosphate and calcium sulphate.

Hypoglycemia often occurs after food allergens are consumed, triggering uncontrollable hunger and eating. Any food can trigger hypoglycemic symptoms and any system in the body can be affected, but most sensitive people have a target organ. Once the pancreas has become hypersensitive to sugar over a long period of time, complete recovery is not always possible. In experiments with rats who were fed refined carbohydrates until clinical hypoglycemia developed, it was found that hypoglycemia could be corrected and kept under control with a change in diet. If the old diet was reverted to then hypoglycemia and the resulting symptoms returned fairly rapidly. Obviously your child is not a rat, but the lesson is there. A more healthful diet will undoubtedly improve your child's health.

Chapter 11

⌐

ESSENTIAL FATTY ACIDS

Uring the past century or so, the amount of total fat in our diet has nearly doubled due to the inclusion of margarine and highly processed vegetable oils. These oils did not exist before 1800. Manufacturers now want products that last indefinitely on the shelves of grocery stores. They have introduced oils that contain unnatural and unhealthy substances, as well as fats and oils that are deficient in the essential components.

WHAT ARE EFAS?

While most fats are recognized as being bad for health, there are some fats that are necessary for health. These are the essential fatty acids (EFAs). EFAs function as building blocks in the membranes of every cell in the body. About twenty specific fatty acids are required by the human body to maintain normal function. The body can make all of them but two—Omega-3 (linolenic acid) and Omega-6 (linoleic acid). These must be obtained from the diet or from supplements.

Omega-3 and Omega-6 oils are both necessary for the healthy functioning of the body, especially for the heart, brain, and cell membranes. They are the precursors of substances that regulate many body functions, including the immune system and the ability to fight infection. They also help maintain body temperature, insulate nerves, cushion and protect the tissues, and are vital to metabolism. They promote adrenal hormone production, skin and hair health, make calcium available for tissue use, elevate the calcium level of the bloodstream, and aid in weight reduction by burning saturated fats.

An unborn child requires Omega-3 fatty acids for the development of the brain and to form the membranes that protect cells from invasion. Essential fatty acids are exactly that—essential. Life without them is impossible and when you have a deficiency you can expect health problems. The average person now receives only a fraction of the "good" fats that were present in the diet of our ancestors. A deficiency can lead to an astonishing array of physical problems, including the symptoms of ADD.

ADD AND EFA DEFICIENCY

The Hyperactive Children's Support Group in England has researched and found the connection between ADD and the deficiency of essential fatty acids. Their research has led them to suspect that hyperactive children might have a problem with an important pathway in the body that converts EFAs to prostaglandins—tissue-like hormones that control all bodily functions at the cellular level. The group's survey reveals that many children cannot metabolize nor absorb EFAs normally. The EFA requirements of these children are thus higher than normal. An EFA deficiency results in some serious symptoms—many of which look like ADD. Other common symptoms are eczema, asthma, and allergies.

The following points suggest the involvement of EFAs in ADD-like behavior:

- Hyperactive male children outnumber females by three to one. They required two to three times more EFAs than females to prevent the signs of essential fatty acid deficiency. Supposedly, boys have more difficulty converting EFAs to prostaglandins.
- About two-thirds of children with EFA deficiencies have abnormal thirst. Thirst seems to be a key feature.
- Asthma, eczema and other skin problems are more common in hyperactive children. This is because of the defective formation of prostaglandins.
- Many children with ADD are zinc deficient. Zinc is required for the conversion of EFAs to prostaglandins.
- Wheat and milk can adversely affect some children. These foods can block the conversion of EFAs.

Fatty acids must be converted in order to be used. Diet plays a key role in the process because it takes adequate zinc, vitamin E, vitamin C, niacin, and pyridoxine (B-6) to convert Omega-6 fatty acids to Omega-3 fatty acids. Other factors that can interfere with this important conversion process are chronic illness, stress, and eating large quantities of saturated fats and hydrogenated oils.

The finding that hyperactive children have an EFA deficiency correlates perfectly with the Feingold diet. Dr. Ben Feingold describes a large number of natural food substances and non-natural food additives that may precipitate symptoms in children with ADD. These include natural salicylates and other coloring materials. Many of the agents described by Dr. Feingold are known inhibitors of the conversion of EFAs to prostaglandins, or are chemically related to such known inhibitors.

One of the worse offenders is yellow dye. It inhibits prostaglandin formation when essential fatty acid levels are very low, but has little or no effect when essential fatty acid levels are high. This suggests the possibility that children with normal levels of EFAs are not affected. Adding EFAs to the diet of children with hyperactivity may be necessary to correct the symptoms.

WOULD ONLY ONE SIBLING HAVE SYMPTOMS?

Some families have only one child with hyperactivity, while other siblings eat exactly the same diet and appear normal. There may be a deficiency or a defect in essential fatty acid absorption in the hyperactive child causing him or her to need a much larger amount.

CIS-FATTY ACIDS AND TRANS-FATTY ACIDS

When polyunsaturated oils are hydrogenated and heated at high temperatures, they form into oils called trans-fatty acids. Natural plants have their oils in a "cis" formation, but chemically altered oils have a "trans" configuration. This type of configuration was not a part of the diet in the past. Trans-fatty acids are harder to metabolize and cannot be used in the synthesis of many hormones and important chemicals the way natural fats can.

Good quality cis-configuration oils play an important role in a well-balanced diet. They provide the EFAs the body needs to protect cell membranes and form prostaglandins. Highly unsaturated EFAs (such as flaxseed oil) combined with high-quality proteins work to counteract toxic and poisonous accumulations in all body tissues. Understanding the benefits of EFAs is understanding that the body has many healthy uses for good quality fats.

Fats of bad quality, on the other hand, are extremely detrimental. Trans-fatty acids change the permeability of cell membranes, disrupt the vital functions of the EFAs, and interfere with certain enzymes needed to detoxify insecticides. They can increase EFA deficiency by interfering with their transformation into other important molecules.

WHAT FOODS CONTAIN TRANS-FATTY ACIDS?

We get trans-fatty acids mostly from margarines and shortenings made from partially hydrogenated vegetable oils. Hydrogenation uses strong chemicals that remove most of the vitamins and mineral from the product and results in many altered, unnatural substances that interfere with normal biochemical processes. In Holland, it is prohibited by law to sell margarine containing trans-fatty acids, but in the U.S. hydrogenated margarines and shortenings are found in most processed foods—bread, rolls, crackers, pies, pretzels, cookies, donuts, bread sticks, muffins, bread crumbs, stuffing, pop tarts, biscuits, pancake mix, quick breads, potato chips, candy bars, non-dairy creamers, peanut butter, salad oils, fast-food shakes, baked and canned goods, packed-in-oil products, and fried foods at restaurants. The annual consumption of trans-fatty acids is almost twice as much as the total intake of all other unnatural food additives put together.

AGELESS FOODS AND LOST NUTRIENTS

Manufacturers continue to use hydrogenation because it keeps their product from spoiling for months. What they do not acknowledge is that the nutrients lost during the hydrogenation process are the very ones that are most necessary. For this reason it is best to avoid hydrogenated or partially hydrogenated vegetable oils.

Agricultural methods have also decreased our intake of EFAs. Caged chickens and their eggs, as well as feed-lot-raised cattle, are producing much lower levels of Omega-3 and Omega-6 fatty acids than their free-range counterparts. The same has happened to fish. In the wild, fish eat other small fish, shrimp, algae, insects, and insect larvae that are high in EFAs. Now fish are being farmed and fed soy meal and other less nutritious foods.

In our diets today there has been a substantial increase in drugs and pharmaceuticals, sugar, caffeine, alcohol, and refined carbohydrates that block EFAs and their conversion to the vital prostaglandins. Add to this mix the increase in toxic food, water, and air, plus the lack of breast feeding, and it is clear that the average diet is just not going to contain enough EFAs unless a concerted effort is made to find good quality sources. Not only are we not eating enough of the right types of essential fats and oils, but we are increasing our intake of the harmful ones. For the good of our children, and for our own health, we have got to start making some changes.

SOURCES OF EFAS

Because fatty acids are extremely perishable and quickly become rancid, it is best to obtain them from fresh foods such as cold-water fish (Omega-3) and leafy green vegetables (Omega-6). Omega-6 fatty acids are abundant in other plant sources such as the seeds of sesame and sunflowers and their oils. Other products containing high levels of Omega-6 fatty acids are borage oil, evening primrose oil, and black currant oil. Omega-6 is also present in safflower and corn oil, as well as in walnuts, almonds, tofu, avocados, barley, cashews, garbanzo beans, peanut butter, and rice.

There are two major sources of Omega-3 fatty acids. Fish oils, especially cold-water fish such as salmon, mackerel, halibut, albacore tuna, cod, and sardines, are an excellent source. The richest plant source is fresh-pressed organic flaxseed oil that contains 50 to 60 percent of Omega-3 by weight and approximately 20 percent Omega-6 fatty acids. This oil contains almost twice as much Omega-3 as fish oils. When using flaxseed oil remember that it becomes rancid when exposed to light, oxygen, and high temperatures. Other good sources of Omega-3 fatty acids are nuts, pumpkin seeds, walnut oil and walnuts, wheat-germ oil, soybean oil, soybean lecithin, tofu, common beans, seaweed, safflower and canola oils, avocados, barley, cashews, garbanzo beans, and corn.

FLAXSEED OIL

Flaxseed oil contains both Omega-6 and Omega-3 fatty acids. The suggested dosage is from one to two tablespoons of raw flaxseed oil daily. Use it in salad dressings, pour it over vegetables and potatoes, or take it in capsules. You could grind two tablespoons of flaxseeds in a coffee grinder and mix them with juice, water, soy milk, rice milk, or add to food. The seed mixture will thicken quickly so drink or eat the combination soon.

In order for the Omega-3 fatty acids in flaxseed oil to unfold properly, the other essential nutrients (proteins, vitamins and minerals) must also be present in the diet in adequate amounts. Vitamin B-6 and magnesium must be present for the body to convert EFAs into the beneficial end products. Dr. Donald Rudin, co-author of *The Omega-3 Phenomenon,* believes that a deficiency of Omega-3 oils is partially responsible for widespread illnesses, including the increase in emotional and behavior disorders.

WHAT ARE EPA AND DHA?

Eicosapentaenoic acid (EPA) and docosahexaenoic acid (DHA) belong to a particular class of polyunsaturated fatty acids. EPA and DHA are associated with clean arteries and the absence of fatty degeneration diseases. They can both be produced by the healthy human body from Omega 3 fatty acids, but they are produced very slowly. They are essential as structural components of all cell walls, necessary for proper brain and eye development, and required for the proper functioning of the immune, reproductive, respiratory, and circulatory systems. They are also precursors to prostaglandins, which are also essential for overall health.

EPA and DHA can be found in fish oils. There is not a reliable vegetarian source of the two acids. Claims have been made that it is available from vegetable oils such as flaxseed oil, but research shows those sources of EPA may not be bioavailable to the body. The best supplemental source is from fish tissues (as opposed to fish liver). The best sources are cold-water fish such as salmon, sardines, cod, trout, and mackerel. Remember that if the fish come from fish farms, the amounts of Omega-3 fatty acids are greatly reduced.

If you take supplements, it is best to divide the doses and take them with meals. Find products that also have added vitamin E to reduce the possibility of the oil becoming rancid. Be careful with products that have vitamin A or vitamin D added, however, because they can become toxic to the body in large doses.

ASPIRIN DECREASES ASSIMILATION OF EFAS

There are various health problems associated with aspirin. For one thing, it inhibits an enzyme needed to assimilate Omega-3 fatty acids. Another problem that occurs when aspirin is taken every day is that little or none of a substance that rids the lungs of breathed-in dust and bacteria is produced. People who suffer from allergic disorders may benefit from avoiding aspirin and other non-steroid anti-inflammatory drugs while taking essential fatty acids each day.

WHICH OMEGA-3 FATTY ACIDS ARE BEST?

The oils derived from the seeds of the black currant and borage plants have much more Omega-3 fatty acid than flaxseed oil or evening primrose oil. However, there is a difference. Only a very small amount of an important prostaglandin is formed from black currant and borage oils, as compared to flaxseed or evening primrose oils.

LOW-FAT DIETS—NOT FOR CHILDREN

Low-fat diets are not for everyone. They even may be dangerous for infants and children. Growth requires the energy of concentrated calories, such as those we get from fat. Calcium and some vitamins require fat for absorption. Even breast milk is high in fat content. Growing children are fast oxidizers and require more fat and oil in their diet than adults. Many children with ADD and hyperactivity are eating precisely the wrong diet for their body type. Parents are being told that all fats and oils are bad and often give the children inadequate amounts. This only aggravates symptoms and speeds up the oxidation rate. It is important to add adequate quality fats to the diet.

HOW MUCH FAT SHOULD BE CONSUMED?

If you followed the U.S. Department of Agriculture's (U.S.D.A.) food-guide pyramid to daily food choices, you would eat 6 to 11 servings of bread, rice, cereal, and pasta. These foods, however, contain few EFAs. If you get the proper kinds of fat, your total fat intake should be about twenty percent of your daily calories. Many experts believe the higher the Omega-3 fatty acid consumption, the better it is. It may not be necessary to increase the Omega-6 levels because there is already an over-consumption of Omega-6 from refined oils and margarine. The average person consumes up to twenty times more Omega-6 fatty acids than Omega-3. A healthy balance seems to be a one-to-one ratio.

STORING OILS

Omega-3 and Omega-6 oils are fragile and easily destroyed by light, air, and heat. Their sensitivity is precisely what makes these oils precious to human health. Natural oils will keep four to six months if properly stored. Safflower, sunflower, and corn oils (polyunsaturates) become rancid more quickly than olive oil (a monounsaturate). The best place to store fats and oils is in a tightly capped, dark bottle in your refrigerator. The only exception is olive oil. It has its own anti-oxidants that keep it from turning rancid. Store olive oil at a cool temperature in a dark cupboard. When the temperature edges up into the 70s or 80s, refrigerate it.

To reduce the chances of rancidity, add vitamin E to your oils immediately after opening. Put a hole in the end of a capsule and squeeze the oil into your container. You may want to buy oils in smaller bottles to insure freshness. A gallon of fine oil is no bargain if you use only a pint in two months and the rest turns rancid.

Flaxseed oil only retains its Omega-3 fatty acids unspoiled for about four months. Light, oxygen in the air, and high temperatures destroy it very rapidly. Once opened, consume flaxseed oil within three to six weeks. The container must not encounter light. Add flaxseed oil to foods just before serving, not before cooking. Heating oils can destroy vital fatty acids.

A CAUTION FOR CONSUMERS

A label that pronounces a product is "made with 100 percent pure vegetable oil" is a signal for the buyer to beware. When making unsaturated fats into saturated ones, most vegetable oils undergo a chemical change. The process creates abnormal or unnatural fatty acids. Not only is the body unable to use them as EFAs, but abnormal fats can even block the utilization of the needed EFAs in the body.

Use caution when buying "all-purpose" vegetable oils. They are usually made from pressed cottonseed oil which comes from pesticide-laced cotton plants. Cottonseed oil is a very poor-quality oil. Many sprayed toxins remain on the seeds after the cotton fiber is removed. Cottonseed oil contains a fatty acid, cyclopropene, that is toxic to the liver and gall bladder and interferes with the functions of EFAs. It also contains gossypol, an irritant of the digestive tract, that can cause water retention in the lungs and shortness of breath. But because cottonseed oil is an inexpensive by-product for food processors, it is often used in many packaged products.

So-called "natural" food oils found in health-food stores are not recommended. Their method of production usually differs very little from that of the highly refined, harmful oils. These oils use the same damaging refining technologies and packaging methods as supermarket brands.

Canola oil is made from rape seeds. Since this seed is often sprayed with pesticides, you need to find a certified organic source. Many companies lack organic certification, but falsely claim organic status for their products. Without proper certification, the consumer has no guarantee of the quality of the products.

WHO MAKES THE BEST OIL?

Natural and unrefined oils contain a little sediment, plus a distinct aroma and taste. For years I thought buying oils in a health-food store gave some assurance that they were good quality, health-promoting oils for cooking and salad dressings. I was wrong. Even some health-food brands have deceived the public regarding the purity, safety, and nutritional value of their oils. Most companies do not make their own oils; instead, they buy them from the same giant corporations that produce commercial ones. These companies bottle them, put on health-food labels that say "cold-processed," and sell the oils at inflated prices.

Be assured, however, that there are three companies in Canada and the United States you can trust. Seymour Organic Foods, Flora Inc., and Omega Nutrition all produce oils that meet the highest standards of quality. Flora Inc. and Seymour Organic Foods distribute truly fresh-pressed, cold-processed, unrefined oils and package them in the appropriate dark glass bottles. There is still some penetration with damaging light rays into the dark amber glass causing a certain amount of rancidity. A black glass container would be a better choice.

Arrowhead Mills distributes the full line of Omega Nutrition oils in the United States. They bottle the oils in completely light-excluding containers. They also produce a full line of organic, fresh-pressed vegetable oils that have both Farm Verified Organic and Organic Crop Improvement Association certification. There is a new butter alternative called *Spectrum Spread*, a non-hydrogenated, non-dairy spread, made by Spectrum Naturals of Petaluma, California. The spread is free of trans-fatty acids and saturated fats. (See the "Resource Guide" for the telephone numbers and addresses of these companies.)

Chapter 12

⊡

SALICYLATES AND THE FEINGOLD DIET

Today there are thousands of children being given drugs to control their behavior. If a child acts like he has ADD, give him a prescription, put him on a drug. But how many children really need medication? Could their behavior be changed in some other way? In the 1970s Dr. Ben Feingold, M.D., developed one of the first natural approaches to true hyperactivity. A pediatrician who taught at Northwestern University, Dr. Feingold was a pioneer in the fields of allergy and immunology. He was also Chief of Allergies at Kaiser Permanente Medical Center in San Francisco.

According to Dr. Feingold, many hyperactive children are sensitive to naturally occurring salicylates and phenolic compounds. Salicylates are derived from salicylic acid, which is used as a food preservative and in the production of aspirin. It was Dr. Feingold's hypothesis that food additives induce hyperactivity. He based this idea on over 1,200 cases where food additives seemed linked to learning and behavior disorders. In 1973, at a meeting of the American Medical Association, Dr. Feingold reported that he believed that salicylates, artificial colors, and artificial flavors in the diet were responsible for 40 to 50 percent of the hyperactive children he had seen in his practice. His statement set off an international furor. Even clinical ecologists were skeptical. How could such a small list of substances be such a frequent cause of hyperactivity?

CAN DIET AFFECT BEHAVIOR?

After years of testing and research, Dr. Feingold published *Why Your Child Is Hyperactive* (Random House 1974). It included a dietary plan to help control hyperactivity. The good news spread quickly. The book describes his behavior-changing diet and the remarkable effects it supposedly had on many of the affected children. Many of the children involved in the studies showed significant improvement in behavior after removing suggested substances from the diet.

Dr. Feingold proposes a diet management plan that adds nothing to the diet, but he recommends that artificial colors and flavors, BHT and BHA, and the flavor enhancer MSG be avoided. His plan includes the removal of many processed foods, other additives, and most of the junk food available. These substances are the most common offenders of the central nervous system. The reason is they contain synthetic coloring and flavoring agents which are the causes of abnormal behavior. They can also cause symptoms of thought-to-be allergies. Any chemical compound—natural or synthetic—can induce neurological problems in an individual who is sensitive to that compound.

As far back as 1940 there were reports of sensitivities to dyes, especially to yellow dye No. 5 (tartrazine). Aspirin and other salicylate substances, naturally found in some fruits and vegetables, contain a chemical similar to this synthetic yellow dye. The chemical name for aspirin is acetyl salicylic acid. Aspirin is one of the primary offenders of the central nervous system, and many other over-the-counter remedies, including artificially flavored vitamin pills, contain salicylates.

More and more, artificial colors and flavors are being associated with health and behavior problems. These include hyperactivity, poor sleep patterns, and behavior and learning problems such as irritability and attention deficit disorders. The degree of sensitivity to any one salicylate can vary from mild to severe. The compounds are fat-soluble and accumulate in the body. A reaction may occur from this accumulated effect.

The elimination of additives in the diet has resulted in dramatic improvement of children who were previously uncontrollable without powerful drugs. Learning problems decrease. It may not be easy to prove this with scientific studies, but the observations of parents and doctors over the past fifteen years confirm that avoiding artificial additives has significantly improved their children's condition. This evidence is hard to ignore. Remember, not every child will respond to this treatment. There are many reasons a child may manifest the symptoms of ADD. Eating artificial additives may be just one of them and you need to address all possible causes. With avoidance of an offending substance, it usually takes less than two weeks to see results. Symptoms usually return immediately with the reintroduction of the additives into the diet. Many physicians are still prescribing amphetamine drugs instead of looking into the possibilities of food and chemical sensitivities.

The idea of hyperactivity being linked to diet has been attacked by a number of government agencies and even some nutritionists. They want more extensive tests of Dr. Feingold's diet. It is interesting that the loudest voice behind most of the criticism is the Nutrition Foundation. This is a group established and funded by the Coca-Cola company, the Life Saver company, and other giant manufacturers of processed foods.

Other studies lend additional evidence to Dr. Feingold's claim that diet is a frequent cause of childhood hyperactivity. A study published in *Lancet* (1985) found that 82 percent of a relatively large group of hyperactive children responded to a hypoallergenic elimination diet. While on the diet, the behavior of many of the children became entirely normal. The most commonly provoking substances were artificial food colors and preservatives. Also included were chocolate, cow's milk, eggs, citrus, wheat, cane sugar, nuts, and cheese. Most children do not react to only artificial colors and preservatives. This may explain why some previous double-blind studies that tested these substances alone had negative results.

An individual may need to make other diet changes if problems still remain after deleting some offending substances. A diet high in refined carbohydrates, especially refined sugar, is a common offender. Some children are more sensitive to additives because their compromised immune system is not capable of neutralizing these toxic substances. Non-food items found in the environment may also cause undesired behavior, learning problems, or poor general health.

THE FEINGOLD DIET

Dr. Feingold's diet eliminates two groups of foods. Group I contains a number of fruits and two vegetables. This group of foods has natural salicylates as part of their structure. You must omit them in all forms—fresh, frozen, canned, dried, juiced, or as an ingredient in other prepared foods.

GROUP I

Fruits: almonds, apples, apricots, berries, cherries, currants, nectarines, oranges, peaches, plums and prunes, rose hips, grapes and raisins or any product made from grapes such as wine, wine vinegar, jellies, etc.

Vegetables: tomatoes and all tomato products, cucumbers and pickles.

If an individual shows a favorable response to this plan, the foods in this group may be slowly introduced back into the diet in four to six weeks. If either parent has a history of aspirin sensitivity, use caution in reintroducing the fruits and vegetables in Group I. An aspirin sensitivity is usually related to an intolerance to salicylates. Try the foods one at a time for about three or four days. If the child's behavior seems normal, add another food item back into the diet. Follow this procedure until you test all the foods in Group I. If these foods show no adverse reaction, you may allow them back into the diet.

GROUP II

If the symptoms continue even with the elimination of foods in Group I, the next step is to avoid all foods that contain artificial colors and artificial flavors. The Feingold plan specifically pinpoints the preservatives BHT and BHA. Do not use any foods that contain these substances. To be safe, even avoid any topical product that contains these additives, including soaps, shampoos, and creams. Carefully read labels. Avoid non-permitted foods for five days if they contain the offending substances. You can have the permitted foods because they don't contain the offending products. When in doubt eat foods that are fresh, whole, and organic.

NON-PERMITTED FOODS (FOODS CONTAINING BHT, BHA OR OTHER ADDITIVES)

- cereals with artificial colors or flavors
- manufactured bakery goods
- frozen baked goods
- luncheon meats
- all turkey with prepared stuffing
- desserts with synthetic coloring/flavors
- beer
- instant-breakfast and quick-mix drinks
- tea (hot or cold)
- oleomargarine or colored butter
- mint-flavored items (toothpaste, etc.)
- commercial chocolate syrup or milk
- colored cheeses
- chili sauce, tabasco, tartar sauce

- all instant-breakfast preparations
- cooking fats
- many packaged baking mixes
- all barbecued poultry
- frozen fish sticks that are dyed or flavored
- manufactured candies
- soft drinks including diet drinks
- ice cream, yogurt, sherbet
- variety crackers
- prepared mustard, catsup, and mayonnaise
- soy sauce if flavored or colored
- barbecue-flavored potato chips
- gin and all distilled beverages except vodka
- cloves

SOME PERMITTED FOODS

The following list contains some of the foods that an individual would be permitted to eat under the Feingold diet. These and any other basic foods are usually homemade or fresh and organically produced so that they contain no additives.

- milk
- all poultry, but not the organs
- grapefruit or pineapple juice

- distilled white vinegar
- all fresh fish
- pear or guava nectar

- homemade lemonade or limeade
- all cooking oils and fats
- mustard prepared at home

- homemade mayonnaise
- sweet butter, not colored or flavored
- jams or jellies made from permitted fruits with no artificial colors or dyes

Group III

If symptoms are still present after trying the above elimination diet, then you will also need to avoid the following foods for an additional five days: avocado, banana, carob, carrot, cayenne, eggplant, grapefruit, green or red peppers, lemon, lime, melons, olives and olive oil, pineapple, pomegranate, potato, pumpkin, and squash.

General Guidelines for a Salicylate-Free Diet

- Keep a diet diary and write down everything the individual being tested eats. Also note any symptoms that occur at the time. In the event an unfavorable behavioral pattern reoccurs, the diet record will show the pattern. Symptoms usually occur within two to four hours. If a change in behavior does occur, the food(s) that were eaten most recently are most suspect.
- When following the Group I diet, avoid any fruit or vegetable on the prohibited list. If you suspect a child may have an individual intolerance to a food item that is not on the list, eliminate that food as well.
- Carefully check all package and container labels. Manufacturers list the term "flavor" or "natural flavor" on the label without stating the actual ingredients. If you have doubts, do not use the product. It may contain MSG.
- To avoid artificial flavors and colors, you need to eliminate most baked goods—cakes, cookies, pies, pastries, and puddings. The most common dyes used in foods are FD & C Yellow No. 5 (tartrazine), and No. 6 (sunset yellow), and FD & C Red No. 3. You can still eat all these foods by baking them yourself at home. Just be aware of which ingredients you use.

- Practically all candies on the market have artificial colors and flavors added. Make easily prepared candies at home.
- The greatest success comes when the entire family adheres to this diet. The initial restrictions (Group I) concern only some fruits and two vegetables. In four to six weeks introduce these foods back into the diet. The continued elimination of additives is usually beneficial to all members of the family.
- You can reduce temptation by not stocking the prohibited foods in the house. The support of family members serves as an added incentive for the child.
- Adhere to this diet 100 percent or it can lead to failure. Remember, a single bite or a single drink of a non-permitted food can cause an undesired response that may persist for seventy-two hours or more. This will interfere with any desirable results. It can also keep a child in a persistent state of disturbed behavior throughout the week.
- When using medication, if it is contained in a colored capsule, only use the powder inside. A white pill is not necessarily a safe color to take. Some white tablets have a small amount of red dye in them to make them look even whiter. Avoid colored or flavored medication. Practically all pediatric medications and vitamins contain artificial color and flavors. Consult your doctor and/or pharmacist to be sure. They can look up a medication to find out its contents.
- Salicylates need to build up in the system before a reaction occurs. You may be able to tolerate a food on a four-day rotation diet, but find it causes problems when eaten daily.
- Check all toothpastes and toothpowders, mouthwashes, cough drops, throat lozenges, and perfumes. Health-conscious stores carry alternatives to additive-laden products.
- BHT is in some soaps, hand creams, and shampoos. Topical substances applied to the skin can absorb into the bloodstream and cause reactions. Remember that some people must avoid artificial colors and flavors throughout their lives.

Many individuals with hyperactive behavior improve greatly after the elimination of salicylates in their diet, if that is the problem. (The Feingold diet would be unsuitable for the management of non-salicylate foods related to behavior disturbances.) While the Feingold diet is helpful for many hyperactive children, it is unusual that it relieves all of the symptoms. A large majority of children have to also stop all refined sugar and any other food(s) causing a reaction. If you suspect your child has ADD, this diet reduces hyperactive behavior in enough individuals to warrant a trial for one to two months.

The Feingold Association researches foods to determine which brands are free of both obvious and hidden additives. This information, along with step-by-step guidance, is provided for members of the association. See the "Resource Guide" at the end of this book for more information.

Chapter 13

PHENOLIC COMPOUNDS AND ADD

P
henolics are aromatic compounds found naturally in foods derived from plants, animals, and pollens. These compounds preserve, protect, color and flavor foods. They protect plants against pathogens and help attract flower pollinators. In fact, you can find these chemicals in practically every food you eat every day. They are a major underlying cause of allergic symptoms, as well as many learning disorders.

Foods containing phenolic rings such as salicylates, coumarin, and phenylalanine are frequently the cause of hyperactive reactions. In one study, 57 percent of people tested with phenolic compounds showed some sensitivity. The immune system of animals that were continuously exposed to the same phenols also became depressed. Even fetal hiccups suggest that phenolic compounds circulate in the blood to the fetus and possibly sensitize the child before birth.

The following is a list of phenolic compounds and other food substances and inhalants tested in a large study. Also listed is the relative frequency of hyperactivity induced by these substances:

• Acetyl salicylate (80%)
• Ethanol (70%)

- Dopamine, Nor-epinephrine, and Histamine (50%)
- Coumarin (40%)
- Indole (36%)
- Malvin, Ascorbic acid, and Gallic acid (33%)
- Sugar, Phenylisothiocyanate, Phenylalanine (30%)
- Corn, Beef, Eggs, Uric acid (25%)
- Cat hair, House dust (25%)
- Dog dander (10%)

Milk contains thirteen different phenolics, making it one of the most allergic foods in the diet. The main route for phenolics to leave a milk-producing animal is through its milk. Animals add a particularly reactive phenolic compound to their milk by eating feed which contains cottonseed. Gossypol, the phenolic compound found in cottonseed, is fat soluble, causing it to be concentrated in cream, ice cream, and other milk fat products. Foods at the top of the allergic list, besides dairy, are tomatoes with fourteen phenolics, and soy with nine. Phenolic compounds are also present in substances such as plastics, paper, and rubber.

Manufacturers select high-content phenolic plants for domestic food production because of their ability to resist disease and insects. The phenolics help to preserve, color, and flavor the plants. The same type of compounds are added artificially when food additives are used to preserve, color, and flavor foods. Common additives are yellow dye, BHA, BHT, and sodium benzoate.

It is conceivable that certain plant phenolics may be the allergic components of pollens, dust, or molds. Phenol, the standard preservative in conventional allergy injections, is itself a common allergen. Phenol has a special affinity for the brain and is known to suppress the immune system. Phenol is a major constituent of smoke, so anything smoked may cause a reaction in some children.

Allergies to a phenolic compound can cause a variety of different symptoms. Some people begin crying for no apparent reason, some become depressed. Others experience abdominal pain, distention, and diarrhea, or other adverse reaction to foods. Smooth muscles may also be affected. This causes the constrictions often seen in respiratory problems, such as asthma. Phenolic compounds appear more generally toxic if natural barriers, or the body's ability to detoxify, is not functioning properly. The more the body is overloaded with toxins and stress, the harder it is to defend itself from these chemicals. Various researchers have concluded that phenolics can also act as cardiac stimulants. This accounts for the accelerated pulse after eating certain foods. Many people react to tap water. It seems that chlorinated water normally contains hypochlorite, a molecule which combines with any phenolic compound to form an aromatic compound that can react in the body. This combining of chemicals can be very toxic to susceptible individuals.

The thing to understand is that when an individual encounters a suspected phenol, the exact same allergic symptom, whatever it may be, occurs again and again. Learning disabilities, hyperactivity, the inability to concentrate, and other behaviors that are often diagnosed as ADD can be added to the long list of problems associated with these compounds. The many varieties of phenols may indicate why children's intolerances vary.

Complete avoidance of the offending food(s) or substance is a possible treatment of phenolic allergies, but many times it is very difficult, if not impossible. Another treatment is to neutralize the problem compound. When a neutralizing dose is given to stop an allergic reaction, a child starts smiling, laughing, joking, and his allergic symptoms disappear. This occurs because instead of becoming desensitized to just a few foods containing the same phenolic compound, the child would be desensitized to the one chemical that is present in all of the foods. Since phenolic compounds are often repeated throughout nature, desensitization to a few main chemicals could reduce most of the symptoms caused not only by foods, but also by pollens and environmental chemicals.

A treatment which neutralized phenols has been successful with infants and children, especially with conditions such as autism, mental retardation, insomnia, bed wetting, dyslexia, hyperactivity, respiratory allergies, headaches, asthma, and abdominal pains.

Investigate the possibility of phenolic sensitivity. Neutralizing doses can be obtained through physicians familiar with phenolic therapy. It may take a while to see the full results of your efforts, so have patience. Many people have overcome serious illness with the diagnosis and treatment of phenolic compounds.

Chapter 14

⌐

FOOD ADDITIVES

dditives comprise a big part of the American diet. The
Department of National Health and Welfare defines a
food additive as "any substance or its byproducts, the
use of which results, or may reasonably be expected to result in,
becoming a part of or affecting the characteristics of food."
Additives do not include spices, seasonings or flavorings. Instead,
they are usually chemical in nature. Approximately 75 percent of the
foods we consume undergo some sort of chemical alteration.
Consumers use more than 100 million pounds a year of approved
food additives. In the United States, there are over 10,000 food and
chemical additives legally allowed into our food supply. The average
American eats about fourteen pounds of additives a year and about
eight pounds of salt. Changing lifestyles in this century have resulted
in more additives than former generations could imagine.

SCIENTIFIC STUDIES DONE WITH ADDITIVES

It is true that food additives provide us with a greater selection of
food throughout the year. They add variety and convenience to
shopping. Yet, scientific discoveries indicate these "approved" addi-

tives can and do cause reactions. It appears that young, developing nervous systems are particularly prone to the damage or irritation that many food additives can cause. One effect is excessive activity. Because of this hyperactivity, children are more prone to accidents. There may be difficulties with speech, balance, and learning, even if the child has a high IQ. Studies corroborate the theory that food dyes can affect behavior and learning in some children. According to Dr. Ben Feingold, more than 50 percent of hyperactive children are sensitive to artificial food colors, preservatives, flavors, and to naturally occurring salicylates and phenolic compounds. He based his claims on over 1,200 initial cases of learning and behavior disorders that improved significantly when food additives were eliminated from the diet.

Additives are receiving more attention from scientists on a worldwide basis as a cause of adverse reactions. A recent study conducted at the Royal Children's Hospital, University of Melbourne, Australia, determined that synthetic food coloring had an effect on behavior in hyperactive children. In a six-week trial, 200 children were given a diet free of all synthetic food coloring. The parents of 150 children reported significant behavioral improvement. They noted that children's behavior worsened when foods containing artificial colors were introduced back into the diet. The more synthetic food coloring the children consumed, the longer the undesirable behavior lasted.

In the Australia study, behavioral changes associated with the intake of yellow dye included irritability, restlessness, and sleep disturbances. The more dye ingested the longer the reaction time lasted. Younger children, ages two to six, experienced constant crying, tantrums, irritability, restlessness, and severe sleep disturbances. The older children, ages seven to fourteen, were irritable, aimlessly active, lacking in self-control, whiny and unhappy. Although other dyes were not studied, their effects are probably similar because the other dyes are also chemically derived from coal tars and have related chemical structures. Interestingly, the children who reacted to yellow dyes had allergies of one kind or another: asthma, eczema, allergic runny nose. They also tested positive for one or more of eight common food allergens. Most of the children studied had members of the family who also had allergies.

In 1979, the public schools of New York City ranked in the 39th percentile on standardized achievement test scores. In an attempt to improve student performance, the sugar content of foods served in the school feeding programs was greatly reduced and two synthetic food colorings were banned. Soon after, the achievement test scores soared to the 47th percentile nationally. Next, all synthetic colorings and flavorings were removed from the food program. The test scores increased to the 51st percentile. With the removal of the preservatives BHA and BHT, the test scores rose even further up to the 55th percentile. Just by changing and improving the food program in 803 public schools, there was an academic improvement of 16 percent.

Consumer Information

In order to avoid the problems often associated with food additives, consumers need to be better informed. What we need is better label information concerning specific naming of additives in foods. Beware of labeling that says "pure and natural." This does not mean the product is additive-free. Most of the coloring in food comes from artificial chemicals. White sugar looks bright and pure because it's bleached. Meat looks healthier and sells better with the addition of red dye. Smoke flavor is actually pyroligneous acid, but the FDA allows food manufacturers to call it "smoked." Less formidable names of chemicals are substituted whenever possible.

Beware that unintentional additives such as pesticides and herbicides remain on plant crops and that hormones and antibiotics given to animals are present in the milk and meat we eat. You will never find these pesticides, herbicides, hormones, and antibiotics on any food label. Don't forget the most popular food additives, sugars and salt. They should always be consumed with discretion. People have a misconception that additives are safe just because the FDA approves them. Did you know that the FDA offers no guarantees for the safety of additives in our foods?

CATEGORIES OF FOOD ADDITIVES

Additives fall into two categories: those that prevent food from going bad, and those that make food more appealing. The following is a list and description of some commonly found food additives that cause reactions.

ARTIFICIAL COLORINGS

Artificial food colors alter the functioning, either permanently or temporarily, of the nervous and muscular systems. Food dyes reduce the ability of nerves and muscles to respond to signals from other nerves. At the same time the intensity of signals sent spontaneously from nerves to muscles is greatly increased. Animal studies indicate that certain food dyes interfere with chemical communication in the brain and normal development. This adds further support to the theory that artificial colorings cause hyperactivity and behavioral disturbances in children (*News & Features*, March 1981, NIH).

The only purpose of artificial colorings is to add color to our food. There are no claims made that they do anything else, and as a result, are not essential. More than 90 percent of the food colorings now in use are coal-tar derivatives. That means they come from petroleum. They are found in jams, jellies, fruit drinks, ice cream, pickles, processed meat, and fish. Caramel color and flavoring do not require certification, but must be labeled "artificially colored" or "flavored." The following list identifies seven of the most offensive colorings:

• *FD&C Blue No. 1* is a coal-tar derivative used as a coloring in bottled soft drinks, desserts, gelatin, ice cream, ices, dry drink powders, candy, confections, bakery products, cereals, and puddings.

• *FD&C Citrus Red No. 2* can damage internal organs and is a weak cancer-causing agent. This red dye colors the skin of some Florida oranges.

• *FD&C Green No. 3* is a coloring used in mint-flavored jelly, frozen desserts, gelatin desserts, candy, confections, baking products, and cereals. It may cause allergic reactions.

• *FD&C Red No. 3* is a coal-tar derivative used in canned fruit cocktail, fruit salad, cherry pie mix, maraschino cherries, gelatin desserts, ice cream, sherbets, candy, confectionery and bakery products, cereals, and puddings. It may interfere with the neurotransmitters in the brain.

• *FD&C Yellow No. 5* (tartrazine) is a coal-tar derivative used as a coloring in prepared breakfast cereals, imitation strawberry jelly, bottled soft drinks, gelatin desserts, ice cream, sherbets, drink powders, candy, confections, bakery products, spaghetti, and puddings. Food manufacturers add tartrazine to almost every packaged food, even though they are probably aware that about half of all aspirin-sensitive people, plus up to 100,000 other individuals, are sensitive to this dye. Life-threatening asthmatic symptoms are possible. This yellow dye is in about 60 percent of both over-the-counter and prescription drugs. You will find it in some antihistamines, antibiotics, steroids, and sedatives. A product does not have to appear yellow to contain this dye.

The average daily consumption of dyes is fifteen milligrams, of which 85 percent is tartrazine. Among children, consumption is usually higher. Tartrazine can promote zinc deficiency. A recent study determined that tartrazine affects behavior in some children and causes hyperactivity.

• *FD&C Yellow No. 6* (sunset yellow) is a coal-tar dye used as coloring in carbonated drinks, gelatin desserts, dry drink powders, candy, and confectionery products that do not contain oils and fats. This dye is also in bakery products, cereals, puddings, and tablets.

• *FD&C Lakes* are pigments prepared by combining FD and C colors with a form of aluminum or calcium that makes the colors insoluble. Manufacturers use FD & C Lakes for dyeing egg shells and other products that are adversely affected by water. Confection and candy products commonly contain these pigments.

Avoid those foods that list colors with numbers, by name, or simply state "artificial color." Colorings can be found in products you would never suspect. I have found red dye in white-colored items to make them look brighter. Yellow dyes are often used in baked goods and cake mixes so that buyers thinks they're getting a product made with eggs.

Are there natural colors that are acceptable? Annatto is a natural yellow color found in cheeses, butter and other products. Beta-carotene is also a yellow color used in some products. Carmine is a natural red color. Some manufacturers use spinach and beet powders to color pasta. Read the label of every food you buy.

ASPARTAME

The marketed names of aspartame are NutraSweet and Equal. Aspartame is an artificial sweetener about 200 times sweeter than sucrose. It intensifies the taste of other flavors and sweeteners. More than half of the people in this country currently consume aspartame—an easy thing to do since it is found in more than 4000 products. The FDA has recently approved aspartame for use in baked goods. More than 80 percent of all complaints about foods and additives previously received by the FDA concerned aspartame products. About 6,000 consumers reported their health problems to this agency, including hundreds of instances of convulsions. Large amounts consumed over time can upset the amino acid and neurotransmitter balance in our bodies. A recent study found that memory loss attributed to diabetes was caused by aspartame.

BHA

Butylated hydroxyanisole (BHA) is an antioxidant and preservative used in many products, including various drinks, chewing gum, ice cream, ices, candy, baked goods, gelatin desserts, soup bases, potatoes, potato flakes, dry breakfast cereals, dry yeast, dry mixes for desserts, lard, shortening, dry sausage, and shortenings. BHA affects liver and kidney function. Many people have allergic reactions to this product and it has been associated with behavior problems in children.

BHT

Butylated hydroxytoluene (BHT) is an antioxidant that is chemically similar to BHA, but may be more toxic to the kidneys. Similar in use to BHA, BHT retards rancidity in frozen and fresh pork sausage, and freeze-dried meats. Food processors add it to potato and sweet potato flakes, enriched rice, and dry breakfast cereals. The base product used for chewing gum contains BHT. You can find it in shortenings and animal fats. Allergic reactions and enlargement of the liver have been the result of eating foods containing BHT. There is a link between hyperactivity and other behavior disturbances in children. England prohibits the use of this food additive.

CAFFEINE

Caffeine is a naturally occurring ingredient in coffee, cola, mate leaves, and tea. It is a flavor used in cola and root-beer drinks. Caffeine is a central nervous system, heart, and respiratory stimulant. It can cause nervousness, insomnia, irregular heartbeat, and noises in the ear. Caffeine can affect blood sugar release and uptake by the liver. The FDA asked for studies on the long-term effects of this additive to determine whether it causes other health problems.

CARRAGEENAN

Carrageenan is an Irish moss derivative with a seaweed-like odor and salty taste. It acts as a stabilizer and emulsifier in chocolate products, chocolate-flavoring drinks, chocolate milk, pressure-dispensed whipped cream, syrups for frozen products, French dressing, confections, evaporated milk, cheese spreads and cheese foods, ice cream, and artificially sweetened jellies and jams. Some uncertainties now exist with this product requiring that additional studies be conducted. While these tests are being conducted, carrageenan is still being allowed in foods.

MSG

The most common flavor enhancer added to foods is monosodium glutamate (MSG). Flavor enhancers usually add no flavor of their own to foods, but heighten or modify existing flavor. More than 75 percent of the population may react to MSG. Snack foods, soups, canned tuna, and many of the prepared foods now found on grocery store shelves contain MSG.

An ingredient listed as "natural flavoring" can actually be MSG. The label doesn't have to call it MSG. There are several names being used on labels today including sodium caseinate, autolyzed yeast, hydrolyzed vegetable protein, or hydrolyzed yeast. Other names are calcium caseinate, textured protein, yeast food, hydrolyzed protein, yeast extract, natural chicken or turkey flavoring, natural flavoring, hydrolyzed yeast, and other spices.

Larger amounts of MSG can cause mild states of intoxication. Its use can also result in a state of uneasiness with a flushed face and a clouded mind. Symptoms from MSG are often called "Chinese restaurant syndrome" even though MSG is commonly used in most restaurants. Symptoms also include a fast-beating heart, cold sweat, headaches, chest pains, weakness, burning sensations, numbness, fatigue, retinal deterioration, and asthma-like conditions. High levels of MSG can affect young children. Studies have indicated that the damage done at the time of initial exposure may not produce any obvious outward effects. Later in a child's development there may be signs of learning disability or emotional instability. To avoid this risk, eliminate all food and drinks that contain MSG.

NITRITES OR NITRATES

Nitrites will prevent the development of some bacteria and add a pink color to delicatessen meats. Nitrites and nitrates are common additives in processed meat and preserved poultry. Food manufacturers add nitrite to 60-65 percent of all pork products in the United

States. They add it to other meats, poultry, fish, and cheese. It is especially common in processed bacon, sausage, luncheon meats, and hot dogs.

ORRIS ROOT EXTRACT

Orris root extract causes frequent allergic reactions. It is used in chocolate, fruit, nuts, vanilla, drinks, ice cream, ices, candy, baked goods, gelatin desserts, and chewing gum.

PHOSPHATES

Phosphates prevent the physical and chemical changes that affect the color, flavor, texture, or appearance of food. There are phosphates in carbonated drinks, baked goods, cheese, canned meats, dry cereals, cola drinks, and powdered foods. Phosphates attract the trace minerals in foods and then continue to remove them from the body. Widespread use has led to dietary imbalances, especially calcium deficiencies.

SODIUM BENZOATE

Sodium benzoate is a flavoring and preservative in margarine, bottled soft drinks, maraschino cherries, dry drink mixes, dry soup mixes, salad dressings, condiments, snack foods, gum, and sauces. Ice used to preserve fish may contain sodium benzoate. It can cause intestinal upset.

SORBATE

Sorbate is a preservative and fungus preventive used in drinks, baked goods, chocolate syrups, soda-fountain syrups, fresh fruit cocktail, some deli salads, cake, cheesecake, pie fillings, and artificially sweetened jellies and preserves.

SULFITES

Sulfites appear on the labels of packages with names such as sulfur dioxide, sodium sulfite, sodium and potassium bisulfite, and sodium and potassium metabisulfite. They are preservatives and bleaching agents used in ale, wine, beer, and sliced fruit. Sulfites are commonly found in shellfish products, soups, wine vinegar, packaged lemon juice, avocado dip, maraschino cherries, potatoes, salad dressings, sauces and gravies, corn syrup, and dehydrated potatoes. Fresh, peeled, frozen, canned, or dried vegetables contain this preservative. They can be in jams, jellies, molasses, marmalades, stuffing, fruit juices, and tomato paste.

The primary use of sulfites is to prevent or reduce discoloration of light-colored fruits and vegetables, such as dried apples and dehydrated potatoes. They allow vegetables and fruits to look fresh even when quite old and stale. Sulfites prevent rust and scale in the boiler water that comes in contact with food. Lemon juice in your tea or splashed on your salad could be a source of sulfites. Fresh-squeezed lemon is okay, but bottled lemon juice often contains sodium bisulfite.

The FDA prohibits the use of sulfites in foods that are important sources of thiamine (vitamin B1), such as enriched flour, because sulfites destroy this nutrient. This additive also destroys vitamin A. Problems range from stomach aches, difficulty breathing, to hives. Some people had fatal allergic reactions to sulfites, especially asthmatics. Now, restaurants seldom add them to their food items. Sulfites may still be added at the manufacturing level.

Since 1985 hundreds of adverse reactions to sulfites have been reported to the FDA. More than one million asthmatics are allergic to this substance. The FDA plans to propose a ban on sulfites used on fresh, peeled potatoes, whether served in restaurants or sold unpackaged in stores. This ban will include French fries.

XANTHAN GUM

The fermentation of corn sugar by the bacterium *Xanthomonas campestris* produces xanthan gum. It thickens, suspends, emulsifies, and stabilizes water-based foods, such as dairy products and salad dressings. It is an ingredient in packaged meat and poultry products. Gum takes away the thirst mechanism and sends a continuous signal to the stomach to produce acid.

The only way the FDA can know about a problem with additives is through consumer and physician reports. Adverse reaction reporting is voluntary and the FDA encourages physicians to report patients' reactions. Most of the time the reaction is not medically treated because the individual doesn't go to the doctor, or the symptoms are not recognized as coming from an additive. The agency's Adverse Reaction Monitoring System collects and acts on complaints concerning all food ingredients including preservatives. If you experience an adverse reaction from eating a food that contains additives, describe the circumstances and your reaction to the FDA district office in your area (see local phone directory). It is important that you also send your report in writing to: Adverse Reaction Monitoring System (HFS-636), 200 C St., S.W., Washington, DC 20204.

Once you recognize your child's need to eliminate, or at least drastically reduce, the chemical food additives in the diet, you will accept the extra effort willingly. You may have to spend more preparation time with fresh, organic foods than you did with highly processed ones, but the effort is well worth it.

Chapter 15

⊡

Not So Sweet—
Sugar and ADD

Studies have shown that destructive, aggressive, and restless behavior significantly increases with the amount of sugar consumed. Refined carbohydrates also appear to be the major factor in promoting unstable blood sugars. Not surprisingly, they are found in junk food and other products with high sugar levels. If every person experiencing hyperactivity, attention deficit disorder, or related behavior and learning problems tried a food elimination diet, the health of most of them would greatly improve.

Researchers at the New York Institute of Child Development suspected that sugar might be a complication in the treatment of hyperactivity in children. They studied the blood sugar metabolism of 265 children and found that 74 percent did not have the ability to properly digest and assimilate sugar and other refined carbohydrates. When these children were put on a corrective diet that promoted a more stable blood sugar, after only two to three weeks they were no longer hyperactive.

Sugar may not be the only culprit of hyperactivity. Also involved may be the carbohydrate to protein ratio. By increasing the protein intake, the needed amino acids produce neurotransmitters like serotonin, which ultimately has a calming effect. Hyperactive children usually have lower than normal levels of serotonin in the blood.

HOW MUCH SUGAR DO WE EAT?

It used to be only the rich who could afford the luxury of sugar, but by 1840 the sugar pushers were handing out free samples. Today, the American sugar industry has the largest advertising in the world, essentially making us a land of "sugarholics." The most common sugar, sucrose, is the white sugar we use at the table. The average American consumes more than 25 percent of their calories as sugars, with an annual consumption of over 113 pounds per person. And this only refers to the consumption of refined cane and beet sugar. It does not reflect the increasing impact of a variety of other sweeteners.

The beverage industry—producers of beer, wine, and soft drinks—uses more sugar than anyone, including the candy industry. These companies consume over 26 percent of refined cane and beet-derived sucrose and about 40 percent of corn syrups used in the food industry. The bakery and cereal industries use about 13 percent of the sugar produced for food purposes.

IS SUGAR ADDICTIVE?

Sugar is one of the most destructive and punishing food items in our diet. It acts very similar to a drug when eaten in large amounts or consumed daily. Sugar can easily cause allergic responses and decrease the ability of the immune system to function properly. If you need a sweetener, it is healthier to use molasses, pure maple syrup, rice syrup, honey, sucanat, date sugar, sorghum, or stevia.

Small children who have not had many sweets usually have little desire for them. Once they get in the habit of having sugar, however, they may begin to crave it. It is not wise to give in to a child every-time he or she demands sugar. Instead, it is better to analyze why the craving is there. Is something else lacking in the diet? Is there some kind of nutritional imbalance?

Those who attempt to quit the sugar habit find they have quite a struggle on their hands. Sugar, like alcohol, is intoxicating. It creates an imbalance of neurotransmitters in the brain. Going off sugar invites withdrawal symptoms with the most common ones being headaches, chills, and body aches. Sugar-addicted individuals often have a family history of alcoholism, diabetes, or both.

TOO MUCH SUGAR—DETRIMENTAL TO GOOD HEALTH

When you eat a candy bar, a piece of cake, cookies, or anything containing highly refined sugar, there is a rush of energy as the sugar enters the bloodstream. This energy is short-lived; in twenty minutes or so, you will probably feel sluggish, tired, cranky, or even mildly depressed. Candy bar ads promise quick energy, and energy is precisely what sugar provides—pure, unadulterated calories. But it doesn't provide vitamins, minerals, or fiber. Empty sugar calories can easily crowd out nutritious foods. If you sip sodas and eat candy but skip on meals, you are opening the door to poor health. Blood sugar imbalances and diabetes often appear after years of sugar abuse. Side effects resulting from sugar consumption may include:

- malabsorption of protein, calcium, and other minerals
- retarded growth of valuable intestinal bacteria
- injury to the pancreas so that it does not provide the proper digestive juices and insulin to the body
- a decrease in the ability to concentrate
- unstable blood sugar
- a decrease in immune system function

SYMPTOMS OF SUGAR SENSITIVITY

Many children are highly sensitive to sugar and most of the sweets in their diet. This is because most children are fast metabolizers. They burn their foods at a faster than normal adult rate. When there is the combination of a fast metabolism and excessive sugar intake, the result can be behavior that is bizarre, anti-social, or even destructive. A high-sugar diet can aggravate other problems, including hyperactivity, anxiety, poor concentration, nervousness, and irritability. If children get aggressive just before lunch, three to four hours after a breakfast of sweet rolls and juice, there may be a blood sugar problem. Some children get headaches after this type of breakfast, others get stomachaches, and still others become hyperactive.

WHERE DOES SUGAR HIDE?

Many foods contain hidden sugar largely as the result of industrial practices that are unfamiliar to the public. A common practice is to feed sugar to animals before slaughter to improve the color and flavor of the meat. The preparation of meat in packing houses and restaurants often involves the addition of sugar. This added sugar is not required to be listed on any label.

Products advertised as reduced fat, low-fat, or fat-free usually have increased sugar in them. When food processors reduce the amount of fat, the taste and texture are also reduced. Hamburger meat may have corn syrup added to reduce shrinkage and improve color, flavor, and juiciness. French fries usually have a sugar coating that turns brown when immersed in hot grease. The batters on fried foods contain some sugar, often sucrose or corn sweeteners. Manufacturers hide sugar in hot dogs and salad dressings, non-dairy creamers, frozen pizzas, and peanut butter. There are hundreds of these "standardized" type foods that may contain sugar without any declaration on the label. These also include canned vegetables, vanilla extract, baby foods, and even iodized salt.

Almost everything on store shelves has sugar in it, even cigarettes. Some foods are even required to have sugar in them by the FDA. For instance, catsup cannot be called catsup if it does not contain sugar. Some shake-on coatings for meat and poultry contain sweeteners. Manufacturers dump sugar in processed foods because they know people like the sweet taste. Soft drinks are the greatest single contributor of sugar to the diet. But there are other reasons why food processors add sugar to their products: the use of unripened fruit in their canned products; the use of chemically grown sweet corn that does not have much flavor or sweetness; and the use of up to 50 percent less fruit in their jelly or marmalade. Sugar contributes to the taste, bulk, texture, and body of many products, and it increases shelf life.

The first ingredient on a food label is the most plentiful ingredient in the product, the second item listed is second most plentiful, and so on. When food processors found out that consumers were becoming aware of the dangers from sugar, they substituted three or four different types of other sugars so that the word "sugar" would not appear on the label, or would not appear as the first ingredient. For example, a breakfast cereal now contains oats, brown sugar, corn syrup, malted barley, malt syrup, honey, and dextrose. Count up—that is six different kinds of sugar. Add them together and they would easily be the most plentiful ingredient in that box of cereal.

Over 50 percent of the sugar the average American consumes every year is from hidden sources. Partly as a result of this, junk food junkies develop large appetites for salt and sugar and then crave and eat more salt and sugar. The best way to avoid problems and cravings associated with sugar is to eat foods that are fresh and not packaged, canned, bottled, treated or sweetened.

IS ONE TYPE OF SUGAR BETTER THAN ANOTHER?

Don't let yourself be fooled by sugar or its many aliases. Sugar, whether cane sugar, beet sugar, or corn sugar, is completely refined and has no nutritional value except for providing empty calories. Sugar in any form is readily absorbed into the bloodstream and provides quick energy to the cells. Sucrose, fructose, dextrose—the body just converts them all to glucose. Glucose circulates in the bloodstream as fuel or is stored in the liver and muscles or elsewhere as fat.

Please recognize that fruit juices are as much of a sweet as candy is—even the unsweetened juices. They are often high in natural sugars, and can have the same harmful effects as candy or other sweets. "Sweetened with fruit juice" sounds like a good thing, but what it really means is that the product is sweetened with juice that is refined down to practically pure sugar. Diets high in juice intake can contribute to a large part of a child's daily calories. The juice replaces other more nutritious foods and leads to a reduction in protein, fat, vitamins and minerals.

How Does Sugar Affect the Body?

To digest simple carbohydrates such as sugar, the body requires additional vitamins and minerals. Eating sugar depletes nutrient reserves, especially the B-vitamins and minerals. A lack of necessary chromium will manifest itself in a sugar craving. This mineral is necessary to maintain a healthy blood sugar level and contributes to the proper use of carbohydrates and fats. Diets that are high in sugar increase urinary chromium losses as much as 300 percent. The more sugar eaten, the more chromium the body loses, which makes the body crave more sugar, and so on.

A deficiency of protein may also contribute to sweet cravings. It is critical that you consume adequate protein, oils and fats. Otherwise you will be hungry and crave sweets. Children deprived of foods such as eggs, avocado, nuts, seeds, and protein-rich foods often crave and eat more sugar, which leads to sugar addiction.

Pediatric researchers at Yale University School of Medicine found that sugar causes a noticeable physiological reaction in normal healthy children. Twenty-five children and twenty-three young adults were given the sugar equivalent of two twelve-ounce cans of cola on an empty stomach while resting in bed. The blood sugar levels fell significantly further in the children than in the adults. The children's adrenaline levels rose twice as high as the adults and remained elevated during the five hours of scientific observation. The body releases adrenaline to counteract the effect of too much insulin and the resulting low blood sugar. The children's brain waves also showed that the ability to pay attention was affected ("Kids Really Do Get a Sugar Buzz," by Jane Brody, *The Seattle Post-Intelligencer*, March 15, 1995).

Complex carbohydrate-based sweeteners, such as organic brown rice syrup and barley malt, are less stimulating than sugar. Natural sweeteners, such as real maple syrup and molasses, don't seem to cause the overwhelming cravings that white refined sugar produces. Two herbal sweeteners that really work well are stevia and licorice. Natural sweeteners also tend to be much less sweet than refined sugars, reducing the likelihood of a sweet-habit developing. Even natural sweets are best consumed sparingly. Remember that any sweet is a concentrated source of sugar. Control your food instead of letting it control you.

DON'T USE SUGAR AS A REWARD

A common mistake made by parents is to give their children sugar-laden foods or drinks, either because children ask for them, or as a reward for good behavior. This can aggravate the problems of hyperactivity, anxiety, nervousness, poor concentration and irritability. You may not see changes in behavior just by giving a child some sugar. Other substances can also contribute to behavioral symptoms. There is often a dramatic difference in behavior and health patterns, both physical and mental, when you withdraw sugar and various chemical sweeteners from the diet. It is not unusual to see ADD get worse when some substances are first withdrawn.

TYPES OF SUGARS

Below is a list of commonly used sugars. They are names you are likely to discover on the labels of processed supermarket foods.

Aspartame is found in more than 4000 products. It is an artificial sweetener about 200 times sweeter than sucrose (table sugar). It intensifies the taste of other flavors and sweeteners. Large amounts consumed over time can upset the amino acid and neurotransmitter balance in our bodies. Symptoms can range from simple to severe headaches, nausea, dizziness, disorientation, confusion, severe anxiety, hyperactivity, personality changes, sleepiness, insomnia, numbness, atypical facial pain, severe depression, slurred speech, convulsions, memory loss, confusion, and other neurological disorders.

Many people with low blood sugar are adversely affected by these sugar-free products. There have been cases of severe reactive hypoglycemia, particularly during the night. Aspartame can make hypoglycemia worse, especially because of the severe caloric restriction and the increased release of insulin.

Aspartame is found in both NutraSweet and Equal. With the use of NutraSweet, symptoms of memory loss, confusion and severe vision loss in some diabetic patients increased. When NutraSweet was eliminated from their diet, vision and memory returned, and blood sugar levels were controlled.

More than 80 percent of all complaints about foods and additives received by the FDA concern aspartame products. With all the adverse data suggesting it has toxic effects on the brain, it would probably be smart to avoid this additive whenever possible. If you can eliminate aspartame completely from your diet, any adverse symptoms can disappear in a matter of weeks.

Brown sugar is the end result of processed molasses. Brown sugar is mostly sucrose and is often more refined than white sugar.

Corn dextrin is a white or yellow powder obtained by enzymatic action of barley malt or corn flour. Milk and milk products often contain corn dextrin as a modifier or thickening agent.

Corn sweeteners include various forms of corn, such as high fructose, dextrose, corn syrups, sorbitol, and mannitol (usually made from dextrose). The use of corn sweeteners is increasing —an average individual will eat more than eighteen pounds per year. More than half the cornstarch processed in this country is used to produce corn sweeteners. Corn-derived sugars are very common allergic substances.

Corn syrups are highly allergic foods and addictive to many people. They can be in maple, nut, and root beer flavorings, and are found in ice cream, candy, and baked goods. Envelope, stamp, and sticker glues contain corn syrup. It is also found in ale, aspirin, bacon, baking mixes, beer, breads, breakfast cereals, catsup, cheeses, chop suey, chow mein, fish products, ginger ale, ham, jellies, processed meats, peanut butter, canned peas, and plastic food wrap

Dextrose (corn sugar) is often sold blended with white sugar. Many artificial sweeteners contain dextrose.

Fructose occurs naturally in many fruits, vegetables, berries, and honey. It is considerably sweeter than sucrose (table sugar). The fructose commonly found in grocery store foods usually comes from cane or beet sugar, not from fruits. It can be very difficult to identify the source of fructose in a food item because of the confusion between fructose derived from fruit or fructose made from high-fructose corn syrups. Fructose does not seem to cause the changes in blood sugar that other types of sugars do. Remember, fructose derived from fruit sugar is still a highly processed sugar, and it does contain calories.

Glucose is a commercially processed sugar derived from cornstarch. There may be confusion with this name because the sugar in the body's blood is also referred to as glucose. The main problem with glucose is its low sweetness level. You could eat a large quantity without being aware of its presence in a food. Ground-meat dishes and luncheon meats often contain glucose, as well as some maple syrups. Confectioners generally use glucose in candy making for several reasons. It gives the hard-boiled candies a clear appearance and costs only half the price of cane sugar. Cheap candies usually contain glucose.

Honey is commonly adulterated with corn syrup or other sugars. To get any nutrition out of refined honey you would have to eat an enormous quantity. There may be contaminants in honey, such as traces of sulfa drugs and antibiotics used to control bee diseases.

Labels citing the source of the honey may not be accurate since bees often visit other plants in the area besides the ones listed on the bottle. A bottle of honey may contain several different blended honeys. Only unrefined raw honey is a nutritive food. This type of honey is getting harder and harder to find. Health-food stores are the best sources for finding this unrefined liquid gold rich with suspended bee pollen.

Malt is sprouted grain, usually derived from barley, or from the hydrolyzed starch of other grains. It forms a thick sweet syrup that is added to foods to improve taste. Barley contains a protein similar in properties to gluten and should be avoided by gluten intolerant individuals. Malt is a major ingredient of malt beverages and non-alcoholic drinks. Most dry breakfast cereals contain malt or malt extract. It is a common ingredient in all-purpose and enriched flour, barbecue sauces, canned and dried soup mixes, caramel flavoring and coloring, cola sodas of all kinds that contain caramel coloring, condiments, salad dressing, milk shakes, maltodextrin, meat sauces, pre-cooked meats, soups, and unbleached flour. The sweet taste in carob candies may come from the addition of malt.

Mannitol is one of the non-glucose carbohydrates called sugar alcohols. They absorb poorly because we do not have the proper enzymes to process them. Mannitol is a constituent of many plants, but is usually derived from seaweed. It digests poorly in the body often causing diarrhea, and can induce or worsen kidney disease. Because it leaves a cool sweet taste in the mouth, antacid tablets, breath fresheners, chewing gum, children's aspirin tablets, and sugarless candies may contain mannitol.

Raw sugar is cane sugar contaminated with so many insecticides, bacteria, fibers, dirt, lice, mold, and yeast that the government classifies it as unfit for sale. All other brown sugars, including ones called "raw," are simply refined sugars darkened with a small amount of molasses or some other coloring agent.

Sorbitol is another non-glucose carbohydrate. Sorbitol can affect the body's ability to absorb and utilize nutrients such as the B-vitamins. It can cause diarrhea if consumed in large amounts. Sorbitol occurs naturally in fruits, seaweed, and algae, but is commercially produced from such sources as dextrose (a corn derivative).

Stevia tastes sweet, but will not stimulate the body's metabolism. This herb's origin is in South America, where it has been used in foods and beverages for centuries. Coca Cola uses stevia as a sweetener when it exports their drink to other countries, such as Japan. To use stevia leaf, simply make a tea (1/2 teaspoon to a cup of water and let steep for fifteen minutes) and add 1/8 cup to a small amount of barley malt or brown rice syrup to enhance the sweet flavor. This combination helps mask stevia's slightly bitter flavor.

Currently, the Food and Drug Administration is trying to prevent the importation and sale of stevia into this country. The American Herbal Products Association (AHPA) has recently submitted a petition to FDA requesting that stevia be granted "generally recognized as safe" (GRAS) status, allowing it to be used freely in various products for consumption. If you would like to support this effort, you can write to your congresspeople, the White House, and the FDA, requesting that stevia be recognized as safe to trade without restriction.

Sucrose (table sugar) comes from sugar cane and beets. Table sugar is refined raw sugar after the molasses has been removed. It is just empty calories, providing no vitamins, minerals, enzymes, fiber, protein, or anything of nutritional value. Sucrose is also a highly allergic and addictive substance. A hidden source of sucrose is the coating for medication tablets.

Sucanat is the registered name for an organically grown granulated cane sugar juice with the water removed. It is unrefined and used in products such as cough drops, candies, hot cocoa, ice cream, and in food preparation.

Total invert sugar is a liquid sweetener more sweet than white table sugar (sucrose). Manufacturers take sucrose and split it chemically and enzymatically to form glucose and fructose. This process is called inversion.

Turbinado sugar is a raw sugar that has gone through a refining process to remove the molasses and impurities. It needs to meet only the minimum sanitary level set by the government. Molasses is the part of sugar that contains most of the nutrients found in unrefined cane and raw sugar. This leaves turbinado sugar with fewer nutrients and more "empty" calories.

Xylitol is a sugar alcohol, just like Mannitol and Sorbitol. It comes from birch trees, corn cobs, peanut shells, wheat straw, cotton-seed hulls, and coconut shells. It has the same sweetness as sucrose (table sugar) and leaves a pleasant, cool taste in the mouth. In high doses it can cause diarrhea. It is still being used in chewing gum.

The main difference between refined sugar and complex carbo-hydrates is that the body tends to burn sugar immediately and may be unable to store its energy, while complex carbohydrates are converted into calories at a much steadier and consistent rate. Refined sugar gives a quick rush of energy followed later by a crash into lethargy and depression. Some people feel that sweets make them groggy and sleepy. Others say that mood swings disappear when they stop eating sugar. Whatever the specific reaction to sugar may be, it is sure that behavior and attention problems are much less severe if sugar is restricted or removed. Understanding this can lead to a drastic reduction in the number of cases that are misdiagnosed as ADD.

Chapter 16

⎏

THE ELIMINATION-
THEN-CHALLENGE
DIET

C ertain foods commonly cause the majority of symptoms of food sensitivities—symptoms which are often mistaken for ADD. When your child avoids the offending foods for a time, symptoms will improve or disappear, but when they eat the foods again the symptoms return. In trying to determine what is causing your child's "ADD" or hyperactivity, this sort of elimination diet should be administered before having him tested by a physician for food sensitivities. Every hyperactive child deserves an elimination diet trial, especially before the prescription of stimulant drugs.

An elimination diet is very safe and cost-effective for evaluating the effect of various foods and food additives on the symptoms of ADD. Your child's symptoms can improve or disappear while on the diet. Then, by challenging the body one food at a time, the symptoms appear and you will know what specific food is causing the negative symptom. Before starting, it is important to decide what symptoms you hope the diet will relieve. Otherwise, it will be difficult to decide whether the diet has been effective. Do not become discouraged if improvement does not occur immediately. The foods causing your child's symptoms can stay in the digestive tract for many days or even weeks. The following outlines the needed steps to take in the diet, as well as lists of "acceptable" and "unacceptable" foods.

PART I

To begin an elimination diet, remove the following foods from your child's diet for at least seven days, fourteen days if possible: milk and other dairy products, wheat, eggs, corn, peanuts, bananas, beef, cheese, potatoes, orange juice and other citrus fruits, sugar, chocolate, coffee and black tea, alcohol, and soy. Your child should also avoid some or all of their favorite foods. Avoid packaged and processed foods whenever possible, as well as canned foods. Your child is not as likely to react to foods that are fresh, whole, organic, and without added preservatives and other chemicals.

Wheat and corn are likely causes of unrecognized food sensitivities and are two of the most difficult foods to eliminate in the diet. Other likely allergens are food additives, especially FD&C yellow no. 5 (found in cheese, butter, and ice cream), pollen, yeast, and spices. Asthmatics should remove avocado from the diet. Eating sugar makes any sensitivity to food additives worse. The following are foods that your child can eat during the elimination part of the diet (unless you know that they make your child ill).

ACCEPTABLE FOODS

- Any vegetable except corn. Beets, spinach, cabbage, cauliflower, broccoli, turnips, brussel sprouts, squash, lettuce, carrots, celery, and sweet potatoes should all be included in the child's diet.
- Any fruit except citrus. Cherries, cranberries (juice), blueberries, apples (juice), and fig are all acceptable.
- Any meats except luncheon meats, sausage, bacon, hot dogs or ham. It is fine to include chicken, turkey, lamb, fish, beef, and pork.
- Any grains except wheat or corn. Include buckwheat, spelt, millet, quinoa, white rice, and oats.
- Any drinks except milk, coffee, black tea, or soft drinks. Herb teas,

mineral water, unsweetened fruit juice (not citrus), and water
are all a positive part of the elimination diet.
- Miscellaneous: It is fine to include nuts, except for peanuts. Honey
  or pure maple syrup can be eaten if a child is not hyperactive.
  Oils such as safflower, sunflower, or canola oil are acceptable. It
  is best if oils used are cold-pressed and organic.

When you begin the elimination portion of the diet, you may
want to add an intestinal cleanser for the first seven days if there is
constipation or the feeling of toxicity.

PART II

On day eight, or when you and your child decide to begin the
challenge part of the diet, select one food that your child eliminated and reintroduce that food into each meal that day. If there is no
reaction to that food throughout the day, you may assume that there
is no sensitivity to it. On day nine remove the food that was tested
on day eight from the diet. Select a new food to test in the same
manner as before. Follow this procedure for each food. Sometimes,
with delayed-onset food symptoms, it can take three days to trigger
a reaction. If the procedure of introducing a new food back into the
diet each day does not work, because you cannot identify which
food is causing the symptoms, then your child may have to introduce a new food only once each week.

Keep a diet diary of the foods introduced and the symptoms.
Start the diet diary three days before beginning the elimination diet.
Continue recording the child's diet and symptoms during the elim-
ination diet, and while reintroducing the suspected foods.

It usually takes about seven days to see improvement on the elimination-then-challenge diet. Some children with chronic food sensitivities won't improve for at least ten to fourteen days. When the
observed improvement lasts for at least one week, you may begin
adding foods back into the diet that you did not think caused any
reaction, but only one food at a time. First, add back the food you
think is the least likely to be causing any problems. Save any sus-

pected foods until last. If the child being tested is sensitive to any of the eliminated foods, then symptoms should develop when the food is eaten again. If you cannot tell which food is causing the sensitivity in your child, here is a suggested schedule of returning foods to the diet:

day 1: add oranges	day 5: add food coloring
day 2: add egg	day 6: add chocolate
day 3: add wheat	day 7: add sugar
day 4: add corn	day 8: add milk

The following suggestions can help make this type of testing more accurate and effective:

• Have your child eat as much of the reintroduced food as they want for breakfast. If there are no symptoms, then your child needs to eat more of this food for lunch, supper, or even at snack time.
• If there is no reaction to the reintroduced food it must be stopped at the end of that day to get ready to introduce another suspected food back into the diet the next day.
• If you think symptoms develop when a certain food is reintroduced into the diet, but just aren't certain, then have them eat more of that food until the symptom or symptoms are obvious. Be sure to keep the rest of the diet the same as before. If there is an obvious reaction after eating any food, then do not let your child ingest any more of that food. Wait until the reaction stops (this may take up to 48 hours) before adding another food to test.
• When adding food back into your child's diet, it is always best to use certified organic ones, if possible, or make sure the food is in a pure form, without added chemicals and additives. Use whole milk rather than a milk product that contains wheat, sugar, and other possible allergic ingredients. A wheat product, such as Cream-O-Wheat, would be better than bread, which contains milk and yeast.

• It is extremely important that no allergic foods be consumed during this test. An accidental or unknown intake of the allergen may precipitate a reaction. Your child must adhere to this diet plan particularly during the trial period. Conclusions derived from this test may be followed for the next several months or years. It won't be helpful if the results of these trials end in false conclusions.

If a food sensitivity is causing your child symptoms, there will usually be improvement after eliminating the food. The symptoms usually return on the first day the food is eaten again. In some individuals the symptoms will not return until the food is eaten in quantity for several consecutive days. If a person eliminates a food for several weeks or longer, there may be a tolerance to that food. Larger quantities must be consumed for several consecutive days before any symptoms reappear. Since more than one food sensitivity is usually involved, there may not be a significant difference if the other foods remain in the diet.

PART III

Once you have tested all the foods you suspect influence your child, you can introduce back into the diet those foods that did not cause any reaction when eaten on a continuous basis. When you test a food that has not been in your child's normal diet, be sure to have them eat it in excess. If your child does not have a reaction after several weeks on the food, do not let them eat that food for four days and then test it again.

If there are obvious, bothersome reactions after eating a particular food, you can shorten your child's reaction time by giving one teaspoonful of a soda mixture. Make it with two parts baking soda and one part potassium bicarbonate. The dosage is two tablets for anyone over thirteen years old; one tablet for children ages six to twelve years; 1/2 tablet for children one to five years old. A laxative, such as milk of magnesia, will also help to stop the reaction by removing the food from the intestinal tract where it is causing problems.

If your child is still experiencing symptoms using the above diet, then continue with the following elimination diet:

- Most vegetables are permitted, but not corn, potatoes, or soy (legume) products
- Fruits are acceptable, but not apples, bananas, or any citrus fruits; this includes fruit-sweetened products
- Meats such as lamb may be eaten, but not beef, chicken and pork
- Grains that are not wheat, corn, soy, barley, or rye are permitted
- Nuts, but not peanuts or Brazil nuts are permitted
- Organic oils made of safflower, sunflower, or canola oil are usually non-allergic
- Only beverages containing bottled spring water or mineral water are acceptable
- Avoid sugar or products containing sugar
- Avoid chocolate, coffee, tea, or alcohol
- Avoid eggs, food coloring, and yeast-containing foods

Avoid all foods that your child eats regularly or more than once or twice a week. If they love a particular food and want to eat it all the time, then be sure to eliminate it during this diet. Avoid commercially prepared foods because they usually contain allergic-type additives and hidden ingredients. Eat simply and buy certified organic foods.

Keep any foods that caused definite reactions out of the diet. After several months of avoidance, your child may build some tolerance to previously sensitive foods, if they are eaten only occasionally. Remember, giving up favorite foods is usually not forever. The symptoms will subside and give the immune system a chance to rest and rebuild. The stronger an immune system the faster health returns. Try to have at least seventy-two hours between the times your child eats the same food, and do not let them eat the same foods two days in a row. Symptoms will usually return if they begin eating the same way as before they began the avoidance diet. Retest any food that does not show a clearly defined sensitivity.

PART IV

Begin to add the eliminated foods that caused reactions back into your child's diet in about six months. Have them eat the food by itself in the morning, before eating anything else. If there are no symptoms it is probably safe to begin rotating the food back into their diet. If they do react, then wait six months before trying the food again. Reintroduction of sensitive foods can produce a more severe reaction than before. Maintain a carefully detailed record describing when foods are reintroduced and any symptoms that occur. It may be helpful to test your child's pulse when you suspect a food sensitivity, since the pulse often changes when a food sensitivity occurs.

A LAST-DITCH EFFORT

If you tried all of the above elimination-then-challenge diets and they do not seem to eliminate your child's symptoms, then you might want to try one more diet before giving up. You will need to limit your child's diet to rice, fish, and steamed vegetables for ten days. It usually takes that long for any foods causing the problem to be eliminated from the body. Of course, do not let your child eat these foods if you know they cause problems. After this ten-day cleansing diet, reintroduce foods back into the diet one at a time as you did before.

An elimination diet may help you detect your child's food allergies and sensitivities, but it is time consuming and requires discipline and motivation. Of course, food sensitivities may not be the problem. Behavioral problems can result from an inadequate diet, or from too many refined carbohydrates. For anyone who doesn't respond to the above program or has very severe symptoms, a visit to a physician trained in food sensitivities may be in order for a more comprehensive program.

Foods that cause violent symptoms must be eliminated from the diet completely. You need to learn which food ingredients may be found in unsuspected places. Avoid all forms of the food. Even the smallest amount can cause reactions. Initially, this may be uncomfortable and strong cravings may occur. Think of these discomforts as withdrawal symptoms. They usually last only a few days and then your child will begin to feel better.

Improperly digested foods set a body up for allergies and sensitivities. Over time there will be an increase in the number of foods causing problems. If your child continues to eat these foods, she will experience reactions with every meal and snack. Continued masked reactions over a long period of time weakens the immune system and can ultimately lead to degenerative diseases and increased infections.

TIPS TO HELP YOU SUCCEED

- You need the cooperation of your child and other family members before starting the diet plan.
- Do not try this diet when your child is visiting others or during a holiday. It is also a bad idea to start an elimination-then-challenge diet when you and your child do not have the time to give it your full attention.
- If your child is in school you will need the school's and the teacher's cooperation.
- You will need medical help before carrying out this diet if your child has a history of asthma, or has experienced swelling or other serious reactions. Consult your holistic health-care provider for guidance.

Chapter 17

⎕

YEAST INFECTIONS AND ADD

Yeasts do not really contribute anything to our well-being, but they are usually part of our non-pathogenic bowel flora. They are harmless when their growth is in balance with other organisms that live in the intestinal tract. If an imbalance occurs, then yeast organisms can become over abundant, leading to established colonies on the skin, in the throat, ears, vagina, as well as in the colon. *Candidiasis* is the medical term for the condition that occurs when the levels of common yeast in the intestines are out of balance. Overgrowth of yeast in the intestinal tract is affecting at least one third of the people in this country, but standard lab tests often don't show anything wrong. *Candida albicans* is commonly the type of yeast that causes problems.

Understanding how yeast can affect us is important because some of the supposed symptoms of ADD may be due to this organism. Yeast can interfere with the formation of fatty acid conversions; it can also overwhelm and damage the immune system, especially when antibiotics are used. An example is the association that has been discovered between recurrent ear infections in infancy and ADD that later develops. Several studies have stated that many of the children being evaluated for school failure gave a history of more than ten ear infections. These children received repeated and prolonged courses of broad-spectrum antibiotic drugs. These drugs alter bowel flora, including the proliferation of *Candida albicans*, or yeast. As a result of these changes, there is an increase in the absorption of food antigens, putting the child at risk for food sensitivities. This may play a major role in causing hyperactivity, attention deficit, and related behavior and learning problems. Problems with yeast imbalance, especially candidiasis, can present unique problems in children, resulting in symptoms and behavioral changes that are not usually seen in adults.

SYMPTOMS OF YEAST INFECTION IN CHILDREN

- Digestive disturbances, including stomachaches, frequent diarrhea or constipation, distention and bloating, gas, irritable bowel, nausea, and cramps
- Behavior and learning problems, such as hyperactivity, learning disability, attention deficit disorders, poor memory, and aggressive or otherwise inappropriate behavior
- Emotional problems, including rapid swings in mood, depression, irritability, anger, frustration, and unreasonable fears
- Muscle problems, including muscle aches, cramps, muscle fatigue, and incoordination of muscle activity
- Sugar cravings or a strong desire for sugar-containing foods
- Allergic reactions, including asthma, hay fever, sinus infections, earaches, eczema, hives or skin rash, runny or stuffy nose, and known reactions to various foods, chemicals or other substances. Problems often begin after antibiotic use
- Urinary problems, such as kidney and bladder infections, or vaginal or rectal itching or discharge
- A generalized set of symptoms that could include fatigue, cold hands and feet, sleep disturbance, blurred vision, itchy ears, and dizziness
- White patches in the mouth (oral thrush) or diaper rash. These

Candida-produced problems will usually clear up completely, but may indicate the tendency for chronic problems later.

DIAGNOSIS

Scientific proof that *Candida* can cause problems like hyperactivity, learning disabilities, depression, anxiety, and various other psychiatric disorders is somewhat limited at the present time. One of the reasons is that there is not a reliable test for intestinal *Candida*. A child's stool can be cultured for *Candida*, but a high yield of the organism may or may not be diagnostic. It seems that the amount of yeast growing in the stool may have no relationship to the number of symptoms the person is experiencing.

Leo Galland, M.D., has found that individuals who have a positive *Candida* culture are less likely to respond to antifungal drugs than those with a negative culture. Evidently, when *Candida* is in the intestinal tract causing illness, the body responds by secreting a growth-inhibitor into the bowel lumen, making the yeast more difficult to culture. People who are not being made ill by their intestinal yeast do not produce this inhibitor, so the yeast is easier to culture. Taking a yeast questionnaire, a good medical history, and a physical exam may be more helpful in determining risk of this organism. A therapeutic treatment trial may be the best way to see if symptoms will clear.

CAUSES OF YEAST INFECTIONS

One of the worse offenders affecting bowel flora and the growth of *Candida albicans* is the repeated and prolonged use of broad-spectrum antibiotic drugs. Antibiotics kill bacteria, both beneficial and harmful ones, but they do not directly affect yeast or viruses. Of all the antibiotics used in the United States, 55 percent are routinely fed to livestock. Nearly all the animals raised for food in this country receive antibiotics sometime during their lifetimes. Eating in a restaurant once a week can increase the risk of yeast infections because of the antibiotics found in the animal fat and dairy products.

In 1994, antibiotic prescriptions for humans posted a record year of 281 million, or 15 percent of all prescriptions. Antibiotic overuse could be making chronic yeast infections into a classic example of physician-induced disease. By killing the bacteria that make up more than 95 percent of the normal bowel flora, the way is paved for yeast infections.

Candida is an organism that usually exists in our lower digestive tract. It also co-exists with many species of bacteria in a competitive balance that keeps it in check, unless that balance is upset. When we are healthy and have a strong immune system, *Candida* is a silent partner and doesn't cause any problems. When our health habits slip into self-destruction, *Candida* growth can continue unchecked, especially in the intestinal tract and the genital-urinary tract. Toxins produced by this yeast will move throughout the bloodstream to all parts of the body and cause a variety of symptoms.

There are other factors that can upset the yeast balance and allow overgrowth. A course of steroid therapy can give the yeast the foothold it needs and sugar in the diet keeps it fed. Poor nutrition, regardless of the reason, can lead to the increased growth of yeast.

FOODS THAT ENCOURAGE YEAST GROWTH

The same foods that commonly upset the human body chemistry are the foods that yeast prefers to "eat": chocolate, most sweets, refined grains, fermented and aged dairy products, dried fruit and fruit juices, alcoholic beverages, pizza, and other refined carbohydrates. When these foods are commonly found in the diet it is easy for yeast to proliferate. Yeast organisms have hearty appetites and they create a craving for more of the foods they eat. It is not unusual to lose the taste for vegetables and animal proteins when high levels of yeast are present, since these foods do not help the yeast thrive. An overabundance of yeast will produce cravings for fermented, pickled, smoked, or dried foods.

What you eat is important, but the way you eat may also be causing many problems. If you have poor digestion, the food becomes a welcome fuel source for the yeast in your lower digestive tract and colon. Along with diet, stress factors add an additional burden on the immune system and make a person more vulnerable to eating the wrong foods.

EFFECTS OF CANDIDIASIS

• Yeast organisms can spread out from the lower bowel to colonize the entire digestive tract, including up through the stomach (especially in cases of low or no stomach acid) into the throat, mouth and nasal passages, and down into the lungs.

• Many people experience adverse food reactions because of abnormal bowel flora. There is a relationship between yeast overgrowth in the intestines and food sensitivities. The bowel wall itself is normally a very sturdy protective membrane that keeps the toxic products of digestion out of the bloodstream. In *Candida* overgrowth, the yeast colonies dig deep into the wall with such a tenacious grasp that they damage the bowel wall itself. The lining becomes inflamed and less efficient in handling food. This can result in allergies and food sensitivities.

Another result is that the bowel walls become more permeable and start to allow large proteins through; in other words, they start to leak. This phenomenon leads to what is called "leaky gut syndrome." It is thought that incompletely digested proteins and toxic by-products of digestion leak into the blood where they cause different reactions at distant sites, such as the joints, lungs, and especially the brain. Other results of a leaky gut may be chronic fatigue, food allergies, immune deficiency, autoimmune disease, inflammatory joint disease, and behavior disorders.

• There are almost eighty different toxins produced by yeast overgrowth. This is a tremendous load on the immune system and could contribute to an increase in other infections and allergies. These toxins make someone feel more sluggish, interrupt vitamin and mineral absorption and action, and cause other body processes to fail. They can affect body hormones and alter nerve transmission, resulting in incorrect signals being sent to the brain.

• *Candida* appears to attack the immune system itself. The immune system goes overboard, producing antibodies to everything at the slightest provocation. This may explain why so many people with candidiasis are allergic to so many different things. It may be one of the major causes of multiple chemical sensitivity. A person with *Candida albicans* has a hard time feeling well without treatment.

DIET AND CANDIDIASIS

The following is a food plan that will essentially starve out yeast. It may help detect food sensitivities as well. On a yeast-free food diet, prepare all foods plainly. They can be fresh, frozen, or canned, without added sweetener. You can bake, roast, steam, broil, or boil the food. Look for antibiotic-free meat and eggs. You will usually pay more for these products, but it is certainly worth it.

ALLOWED FOODS

MEATS
• all meats (fresh or frozen) without hormones or antibiotics
• all seafood
• poultry
• red meat
• game meat
• eggs

GRAINS, STARCHES, AND LEGUMES
• all grains except corn
• sweet potato or yams
• winter squash
• non-yeast breads and crackers

- all fresh, dried, or cooked beans and peas
- tapioca

DAIRY

- rice milk and soy milk are preferable to cow's milk

VEGETABLES

- all fresh, raw, or lightly steamed vegetables, properly washed and peeled (because the surfaces may contain mold)

FRUITS

- limit the intake of fruit; it's best to eat fruit alone and not combine it with other types of food; limit yourself to two servings a day, but avoid fruit juice and dried fruit
- all fruits, fresh or frozen
- melons if washed carefully before cutting open; eat melon by itself
- scrub or peel fruit; the surfaces may contain mold

NUTS AND SEEDS

- most kinds, especially if fresh and raw

OILS

- all oils, but cold-pressed organic oils are preferred

MISCELLANEOUS

- most seasonings without sugar
- most thickeners

SWEETENERS

- none (preferably)

DRINKS (UNSWEETENED)

- herbal tea
- water, especially if purified

SALAD DRESSINGS/CONDIMENTS

• if màde with lemon or lime juice instead of vinegar

FOODS TO BE AVOIDED

MEATS

• barbecue sauces and marinades
• meats if they contain antibiotics and hormones
• cheese sauces on meat
• processed, aged, cured, and smoke meats and fish; includes bacon, sausages, hot dogs, corned beef, pastrami, salami, etc.

GRAINS, STARCHES AND LEGUMES

• malt and malted products
• corn
• yeast (The following substances may be derived from yeast and should be avoided: multiple vitamins, and capsules or tablets containing B-vitamins. Check all vitamin products to be sure that they are yeast-free. Many products that contain vitamin B-12 also contain yeast.)

DAIRY

• cultured or aged milk products such as cheese, buttermilk, sour cream, or sour milk products; avoid dairy products in general

VEGETABLES

• all are allowed

FRUITS

• dried fruit and fruit juice

NUTS AND SEEDS

• peanuts and pistachios

OILS

• peanut oil

MISCELLANEOUS

• vinegar
• soy sauce
• edible fungi (mushrooms)

SWEETENERS

• all types of sugars and sugar-rich foods (see"sugar" section)

DRINKS

• alcoholic beverages
• cider
• fermented drinks (root beer, wine, whiskey, brandy, etc.)
• soft drinks in general
• regular or instant coffee
• all concentrated natural sweeteners
• extracts, tinctures, cough syrups and other medications (that are not yeast and mold, and sugar-free)

SALAD DRESSINGS/CONDIMENTS

• vinegar or vinegar-containing foods such as mustard, catsup, mayonnaise, pickes, and commercially prepared salad dressings
• worcestershire sauce, steak sauce, tartar sauce
• accent, miso and tamari

OTHER TREATMENTS FOR YEAST INFECTIONS

• It is necessary to avoid the foods known to feed *Candida albicans*. A reduction in refined carbohydrates will decrease the source of nutrition that feeds yeast. Avoid foods containing yeast and mold to eliminate any cross-reactions that cause symptoms to flare up and delay recovery. In addition, it is important to eliminate any known food sensitivities at this time. The closer you follow the diet, the better the results.

• The use of an herbal yeast killer containing undecenoic acid is part of the preferred method of treatment. It is very effective with minimal side effects. This herb combines well with caprylic acid to kill the different stages of yeast over-growth. Sorbic and propionic acids selectively inhibit the pathogenic form of *Candida albicans.* There are very effective homeopathic and herbal remedies that help the body regain a healthy balance. All products must be free of sugar, alcohol, and yeast.

• Supportive treatment includes beneficial bacteria. Buy products containing *Lactobacillus acidophilus, Lactobacillus bifidus,* and *Lactobacillus bulgaricus.* These are friendly bacteria that exist in the intestine but killed by antibiotics. These healthy organisms are important in rebalancing the intestinal tract. The acidophilus found in milk and yogurt does not adequately help replenish the intestinal flora, because most of the organisms are killed during the digestive process. Take the *Lactobacillus* on an empty stomach only accompanied by water.

Garlic is a natural antifungal substance, but raw garlic can antidote homeopathic remedies. Vitamin A helps to restore intestinal wall integrity and the immune system. Do not take high doses of vitamin A without being monitored by a physician.

• Nystatin is a drug that kills yeast, but often has side effects of gastrointestinal upset. This is easily remedied by taking the dose with meals rather than between meals, as usually prescribed, or by lowering the dosage. Sometimes it is best to increase the dosage gradually because as the yeast is killed, toxins are released. Symptoms can become worse for a while. Vitamin C helps neutralize these reactions. The maintenance dose is extremely variable between individuals. The duration of treatment is equally variable from person to person.

• It is helpful to use some type of herbal cleanse to detoxify the intestinal system, move the bowels more regularly, and provide an environment for the desired intestinal flora to flourish.

• Remove strong odors and toxic household cleansers from the home because they place an additional toxic burden on the body. People with *Candida* are usually unable to tolerate chemical smells, household cleansers, perfume, etc. Avoid processed foods contaminated with industrial solvents, artificial flavorings, colorings, and preservatives.

• Avoid antibiotics and immune suppressant drugs, such as prednisone and cortisone. If an antibiotic is necessary because of illness, then supplement with a high-count *Lactobacillus acidophilus* and *L. bifidus* for at least a month after you discontinue the drug. Products are available that contain several other types of intestinal flora helpful to the intestinal tract. It is important not to feed the yeast during this time with refined carbohydrates. Treatment of *Candida albicans* requires aggressive action.

A WARNING

Most people view *Candida albicans* as a sort of parasite. They see themselves as the innocent victim of a malicious, opportunistic organism that invades and attacks their body. In reality, we are not necessarily the innocent victims of disease, but often have control over our health. If we pay attention to our body, we will realize that every symptom is a signal—an important message that something in our life needs to change. When we have made the proper changes, our self-healing mechanisms will be free to perform. Our body gives us signals when drugs, foods, and other forms of distress have weakened our defenses. It's our smoke detector, our burglar alarm, our seat-belt buzzer. The signal may be annoying, but the early warning enables us to seek change for better health.

Section Three

THE WORLD WE LIVE IN— LIVE IN— ENVIRONMENT AND ADD

Chapter 18

⌐

ENVIRONMENTAL
FACTORS

For thousands of years, our environment has contained entirely natural foods free from ingredients like preservatives, flavorings, colorings, and refined sugar. Now, many new factors have occurred in our environment. Any significant environmental change, such as chemicals in the diet, unnatural-spectrum lighting, lead exposure, or television radiation, is more likely to be harmful to the health than beneficial. Hyperactivity and attention deficit are only two of the many health problems caused by deviation from a natural environment. We still face many problems. Our departure from natural ways has yet to reveal all the damage possible to our health.

Other factors in the environment may also be responsible. Many children that I see in my office are also sensitive to the chemical content in the air. Our local environments contain more air-borne chemicals, especially in urban and industrial areas. The air is likely to contain a phenolic component or a hydrocarbon (petroleum by-product) that can provoke chemical sensitivities.

Exposure to chemicals may only cause minor symptoms at first. Depletion of nutrients in the body along with continued exposure to these toxins can only lead to illness. Each health complaint gets treated as an isolated ailment instead of recognizing the underlying chemical poisoning that is really causing all the symptoms. If the underlying cause remains untreated, the damage will continue. With the addition of suppressive drugs, the condition that started out with a simple solution has now become a serious problem. To give another chemical to an already compromised system just does not work. It is essential to find the underlying cause.

Donald Dudley, M.D., a physician in Seattle Washington, is researching the brain mapping that occurs in a chemically sensitive person. This new research can identify actual injury in the brain of sensitive individuals when exposed to common chemicals. He discovered that smelling something can directly affect the brain. Chemically sensitive individuals can have a reduction in thinking, concentration, and memory. They may struggle with depression and fatigue, muscle weakness and emotional problems. Being exposed to these toxic substances every day can cause continuous symptoms.

THE "INSIDE" FACTOR

Another environmental hazard is that houses and buildings are more airtight then ever before, increasing our exposure to toxic chemicals. You do not have to be aware of a chemical odor for damage to occur. Carbon monoxide can kill without any knowledge of its presence. Toxic scents are everywhere. They are in cosmetics, household items, detergents, magazine advertising, and body-care products. The majority of these ingredients have minimal testing for human toxicity. In fact, some ingredients are never tested. The National Academy of Sciences reports that 95 percent of chemicals used in fragrances are synthetic compounds derived from petroleum. These chemicals can cause allergic reactions and central-nervous-system dysfunction. Many ingredients found in fragrances are airborne contaminants, neurotoxins, hazardous waste disposal chemicals, and sensitizers. Sensitizers have the ability to cause multiple chemical sensitivities. We really don't know what is in some specific products, especially fragrances, whose companies generally do not have to disclose their ingredients.

Most household products found in retail grocery stores contain harmful toxic chemicals. Many are toxic when absorbed through the skin or inhaled. Washing clothing or bedding in these household products is another source of contact. According to the National Institutes of Health, 35 million Americans experience allergic reactions and hypersensitivity to chemicals found in common household products.

THE "SICK SCHOOL" SYNDROME

Schools are also to blame in contributing to exposure of toxins. Many routinely use products that emit toxic fumes during school hours. The health risk from air pollution is as much as six times greater for children than for adults. On any given school day, your child faces huge amounts of hazardous chemicals. The average young student confronts enough toxic chemicals to tax any liver or immune system. Some of these potent chemicals end up being stored in their body. This includes gasoline and diesel exhaust, paints, janitorial cleansers, designer perfumes, dry-cleaned clothing, polishes, rubber cement, permanent marking pens, aerosol fixatives, herbicides, room deodorizers, floor waxes, vinyl and polyurethane flooring, and pesticides. Carpets will give off formaldehyde, toluene, xylene, benzene, styrene, mold inhibitors, fire retardants, dirt-repellent coatings, pesticides, and other potent chemicals. Carpets also support the growth of mold and dust mites. The flickering lights, chalk dust, and school pets could also be contributing to the problem.

Now, imagine your children in these classrooms and buildings for eight hours a day, five days a week. Imagine them breathing in all these toxic substances. If the school building is more than twenty-five years old, you can also include the asbestos factor. Add to this mix the fast-food diet that your child is eating, and you should not be surprised that your child develops a learning disability. Thanks to modern technology, we have created a world that is making our children sick.

The good news is that a negative environment can be overcome. I am familiar with the story of a school teacher who was also the parent of a child diagnosed with ADD. This teacher counted twenty-six products used in and around the school that had toxic chemicals and pesticides in them. After she brought her findings to the attention of the principal of the school, many changes were made. Natural and non-toxic products replaced the toxic ones previously used. The teacher's child is now doing much better and no longer has any symptoms of ADD. This effectively shows that it really is possible to make a benificial change in a child's environment.

Why is environmental toxin contamination so common? One reason is because the traditional physician does not receive training to detect environmental factors that can change a child's behavior and energy level. An allergy or sensitivity can affect any organ or body system, including the brain. It is very important that concerned parents and teachers educate themselves about classroom dangers, as well as the symptoms they cause. Special workshops can empower educators, parents, and students with the needed skills to make schools safe. These workshops teach how to identify the types of chemicals present in the schools and their potential threat to a student's health and learning. They also help you develop practical strategies to cure the contaminated classroom (See the "Resource Guide" for more information.)

How can you and your child avoid toxicity? Do all you can to purify your home and school environments. Remove any known toxic materials, such as stored or leaking chemicals, dyes, paints, solvents, glues, acids, household insecticides, or cleaning agents. If the toxic materials can't be removed, an effective air purification system may be needed. Regular cleaning or replacement of furnace and air conditioning filters may be also be helpful. Educate the head of your child's school about these toxic substances, and find non-toxic alternatives (they do exist). In this way you can reduce the family's total toxic load.

ELF WAVES AND ADD

There is evidence that ADD and/or hyperactivity may be caused by exposure to electromagnetic fields. Information about the biological effects of long-term exposure to the increased number of electromagnetic low frequency (ELF) waves is being gathered from around the world. Effects include decreased production of dopamine, serotonin, and norepinephrine (neurotransmitters) in the brain, alterations in biological cycles, and increased chronic stress that leads to immune system deficiencies. Children with already impaired immune, endocrine, or nervous systems may have more pronounced symptoms because of exposure.

Behavioral disturbances occur during electrical and magnetic storms. Since humans are electrical in function, they are affected by these fluctuations. Telecommunications, electrical power plants, transmission lines, appliances, microwaves, radar, and radio transmissions have all increased at an alarming rate during the past 50 years. Repeated exposure to ELF waves can cause neurological reactions, such as confusion, hyperactivity, memory loss, sleep disturbances, tingling skin, chronic stress syndromes, more infections, and chronic fatigue. The following may indicate an electromagnetic imbalance:

- Telephone use makes your child nervous, anxious, or headachy
- Watches stop, lose or gain time, or cause sleepiness when worn
- Fluorescent light causes hyperactivity, headaches, or blurred vision
- Symptoms worsen near high-powered electric lines/transformers
- Electrical equipment malfunctions when your child is near
- Adverse symptoms are relieved by taking a shower or bath, or standing barefoot on damp grass

In school settings other environmental factors may affect a child's behavior. In particular, standard cool-white fluorescent lighting increases hyperactive behavior while full-spectrum lights with radiation shields decrease hyperactivity. Our bodies are adapted to full-spectrum white light. This type of light is important to normal brain function and can stop hyperactivity in some children. Behavior studies in school children show that normal lighting can be a factor in hyperactivity and inattention.

Part of the problem is that standard fluorescent tubes emit X-rays and harmful radio frequencies, but do not emit the ultraviolet wavelengths found in sunlight. There are now fixtures available that can remedy this problem, if schools would only look into this possibility. Some people can live in a dark, smoggy city, in a small hovel with artificial light, but this does not mean that all is well. Read the book *Health and Light* by John N. Ott. It explores the effects of natural and artificial light on humans and other living things.

Our bodies have a remarkable capacity to tolerate exposure to harmful substances, but when we are in constant contact with toxins, it can be very difficult to cope. Every day we are exposed to air and water that are no longer pure. Our food contains growth hormones, antibiotics, and pesticides. The processing of food removes the essential fiber and nutrients. Most food advertising directed toward children promotes wrong eating. And the environment is constantly bombarding us with contaminants and impurities. Is there any wonder why children are having behavior problems?

Chapter 19

⌐

HEAVY METAL CONTAMINATION

Numerous studies show a strong relationship between childhood learning disabilities and body stores of heavy metals, particularly lead. The reason toxic metals have not attracted widespread attention is that doctors do not routinely order a heavy metal detection test. This oversight is detrimental to our children because a hair analysis test for heavy metal toxicity, when correctly performed and interpreted, is an invaluable screening tool that could help prevent many cases of learning disability. Over time, heavy metals stored in the hair become a record of these toxic substances. A hair analysis test is inexpensive, non-invasive, and simple to perform. Hopefully, it will become a routine part of every child's physical examination.

Studies done on much of the U.S. criminal population found high levels of lead and cadmium in prisoners during their crime periods. When compared with the general population, prison populations commonly have higher levels of heavy metals. Hopefully, recent interest in the cause of violent behavior will lead to further research on the link between the way toxic chemicals alter the brain and resulting violent behavior. Poor nutrition and the elevation of heavy metals usually go together. Foods that pull the heavy metals out of the body or decrease their absorption are usually missing from the diet. Violent criminals usually have substandard levels of essential nutrients.

Research has found that heavy metal patterns in hair samples can distinguish violent individuals from non-violent individuals. This relationship between heavy metal toxicity and violent behavior represents a significant breakthrough in the explanation of such behavior. A state senator in California has gone so far as to write a bill requesting that a five-year research project be authorized to further research the correlation between violent behavior and abnormally excessive levels of certain heavy metals in the body of criminals and other people exhibiting antisocial behavior.

When it comes to children, the correlation between metal levels and behavior is just as strong. I know of a nine-year-old boy from Washington who became involved in a severe crime. He spent most of those nine years living near a smelter that assuredly gave off various toxins. A hair analysis done on the boy revealed elevated copper and manganese levels and very low zinc levels. These findings are significant because we know that when zinc levels are low, copper can become very toxic to the body. A high level of copper irritates the nervous system and causes a child to be more excitable and to display irrational behavior. Manganese levels of more than .7 parts per million in hair have been another marker for violence in children. The boy's doctor, however, ignored the possibiliy of metal poisoning. After trying eight different medications, he simply put the child on Ritalin. Wouldn't it have been better to find out about the heavy metal toxicity, and then treat the cause rather than the symptoms? Sadly, doctors rarely consider heavy metal poisoning as the cause of behavior problems.

HEAVY METAL TOXICITY

Here is a list of some of the metals that are most commonly found in high levels in the body. Each of them can be toxic and can affect behavior in various ways. Many labs will analyze heavy metal toxicity. You can also find holistic health practitioners who do this type of testing. They also have treatment plans for removing toxic metals from the body.

ALUMINUM

Aluminum plays an important role in health. High levels of aluminum affect the central nervous system and may be involved in hyperactivity and other behavior problems in children. We can easily take in too much aluminum simply because food and water may be contaminated when cooked in aluminum pans or stored in aluminum foil. This metal is found in coffee, bleached flour, antacids, drinking water, and in soil soaked by acid rain. Deficiencies of magnesium and calcium increase the toxic effects of aluminum in the body.

CADMIUM

Cadmium is highly toxic which concentrates in the kidney, liver and blood. It is a neurotoxin suspected of causing learning disabilities. Cadmium is harmful from the very beginning of life—it interferes with zinc absorption and utilization by the fetus. Exposure continues after the child is born since cadmium is found in the air. This can be the beginning of a learning and behavior disorder in the child. Studies indicate that some children with learning disabilities have significantly higher cadmium and lower zinc levels than children without learning disabilities.

Cigarettes are the major source of cadmium in our society. A fetus' first exposure to cadmium can be from a smoking mother. Coffee is the second largest source of cadmium, while white refined flour is another principal source. Zinc used for galvanizing iron (tin roofs, pails, water storage tanks, iron pipes, gutters, nails and a variety of other products) can contain up to 2 percent cadmium. In this way our tap water can be contaminated. Another provider of cadmium contaminants is the zinc and copper smelters and refiners. They release more than two million pounds of cadmium into the air annually. Only a small amount of cadmium absorbs into the body when swallowed, but about 50 percent of cadmium that is breathed can be absorbed into the body.

It is important to realize that the absorption of cadmium from the environment is strongly linked to our diet. An interesting study investigated the relationship between hair cadmium levels and a refined carbohydrate diet in 150 school children. Cadmium levels were higher in the children with the most refined carbohydrates in the diet. This suggests that the consumption of refined, low-nutrient foods increases the body's cadmium burden. Cadmium displaces zinc in biochemical reactions and can slow or halt processes normally catalyzed by zinc. Adequate zinc intake may protect against the adverse effects of cadmium. Once in the body, cadmium is difficult to remove because it has a half-life of seventeen to thirty years. Elimination of this toxic metal from the body is accomplished through nutritional therapy, but this can take six to twelve months.

COPPER

A copper toxicity enhances emotional sensitivity, producing a tendency for mood swings and erratic behavior. Excessive copper displaces zinc in the body. Since zinc is a sedative mineral and a stabilizer of emotions, a deficiency of zinc and an elevated copper level is a frequent cause of hyperactive behavior.

Stress depletes zinc from body tissue. Stress also taxes the adrenal glands. When the adrenal glands function properly, they produce a copper-binding protein. This is another way that stress can lead to a copper toxicity.

Some children are born with these excessively high copper levels. Copper toxicity can be passed from mother to child. Toxic metals are known to readily pass through the placenta. The child acts as reservoir for toxic metals that are difficult for the mother to eliminate. Children who consume junk foods, soda pop and other empty-calorie foods are more prone to copper toxicity problems. This may include hyperactivity, learning disorders, failure to thrive, recurrent infections, and other symptoms associated with a copper imbalance.

LEAD

Exposure to lead is considered the nation's most serious environmental threat to the health of children. Approximately 400,000 babies with toxic blood levels are delivered each year in the United States. One child in six has a toxic level of lead exposure. Among children living below the poverty level, 55 percent have toxic levels of lead. Families with high incomes usually have less toxic levels, but they can occur in expensive renovated mansions. At an annual meeting of the American Academy of Child and Adolescent Psychiatry, Dr. Herbert L. Needleman stated that any child with behavioral disorders or learning disabilities should be tested for lead exposure. He associates even low-level lead exposure with hyperactivity, attention deficits, and developmental failure. The federal government now states that all children should undergo lead testing. A plan for the phasing-in of universal screenings, beginning with children who live in cities and in old housing, is now being worked out.

Lead affects brain function because of its neurotoxic effects, and is linked to a number of neurological and psychological disturbances, including ADD. Screening for lead toxicity, as well as other heavy metals, is an important part of evaluating a child with ADD or any developmental delay or behavior problem.

There appears to be an increase of lead in our drinking water. The Environmental Protection Agency (EPA) found that over 800 municipal water systems, serving 30 million people, had lead levels that exceeded federal guidelines. Water is second only to the ingestion of lead-based paint as a source of poisoning. We absorb lead from water that flows through old lead plumbing pipes or lead solder in our houses. Water can also leach lead from new brass fixtures.

Small amounts of lead can also be leached from glazes and decorative paints on ceramic dinnerware, from lead crystal, and less frequently from pewter and silver-plated hollow ware. FDA scientists found that about 80 percent of lead exposure comes from food which is in contact with ceramic hollow ware. This is especially true of frequent or daily uses of mugs containing hot, acidic drinks. Antiques and other collectibles may look attractive, but this type of dinner ware is more likely to leach lead than those made more recently. Consumers can guard against exposure to lead in food by observing the following guidelines:

- If you are pregnant, avoid the use of ceramic mugs when drinking hot, acidic beverages such as coffee or tea, and avoid the use of lead crystalware.
- Do not feed babies from lead crystal bottles.
- Do not store acidic foods such as fruit juices in ceramic containers.
- Do not store drinks in lead crystal containers.
- Stop using items that show a dusty or chalky gray residue on the glaze after they are washed.
- Follow label directions on any ornamental product with a warning such as "not for food use" or "for decorative purposes only."
- Wine sealed with a foil capsule needs the rim of the bottle wiped with a cloth dampened with water or lemon juice before removing the cork (of course, pregnant women and children should not be drinking wine).
- Have your water supply tested for high lead levels. The use of lead-based solders in modern copper plumbing systems increases the intake of lead through the very water we drink.
- Filter your home water supply with a filter that will remove heavy metals.
- Always wash your fruit and vegetables in filtered water before use. If possible, buy your produce from farms in areas that have low air pollution.
- Don't use any imported canned foods. The cans are often lead-lined.

There are kits to test for lead leaching from ceramics that consumers can use at home. These kits are not always sensitive enough to detect lead at lower levels, but they can be valuable for identifying items that release larger amounts. For information about these kits and other questions about lead, contact your local FDA office listed in the blue pages of the phone directory, or call FDA headquarters at (301) 443-4667. The National Safety Council, under a grant from the federal government, maintains a National Lead Information Center with a toll-free number (800) LEAD-FYI, or (800) 532-339. Also, most U.S. ceramic manufacturers maintain toll-free lines where consumers may obtain information about lead levels in their products. A public affairs specialist in the FDA district offices can provide consumers with these numbers.

The Can Manufacturers Institute informed the FDA that as of November 1991, lead-soldered cans are no longer being produced in the United States. However, lead-soldered cans are permitted in some countries that continue to export canned food to the United States. The FDA estimates that up to 10 percent (some 230 million pounds) of food imported each year may be packaged in lead-soldered cans.

The average adult absorbs 10 to 15 percent of the lead that reaches the digestive tract. Young children and pregnant women, however, absorb as much as 50 percent. This may be because the body cannot distinguish between calcium and lead. Because young children and pregnant women absorb calcium more readily to meet their extra needs, they also absorb more lead. Lead also gets into the blood of pregnant women from their own bone stores. During a period of physiological stress such as pregnancy or lactation, bone-stores of toxic metals can be mobilized back into a woman's blood and increase her blood-lead level. As the blood circulates, the fetus will then pick it up.

Parents bring lead home from the work place and expose other family members. Those who work in construction, torching or sand blasting and have to deal with structural steel coated with lead paint are especially at high risk. There is also high risk if you work with lead paint, recycle batteries for the lead, repair radiators, or have involvement with the demolition of lead materials.

MANGANESE

Toxicity from an overload of manganese in the brain causes a depletion of the neurotransmitter dopamine, leading to hyperactivity. Excessive and toxic levels of manganese are also toxic to the brain's neurons. Three separate studies show an association between high manganese levels and learning disabilities in children. Since infant formulas contain 3 to 100 times the manganese content of breast milk, it is being suggested that these formulas may contribute to an overload of manganese.

The first symptoms of manganese overload are fatigue, a hypnotic-like state or trance, irritability, and erratic behavior. An individual suffering from "manganese madness" may exhibit various antisocial acts or compulsive acts, irrational and violent behavior, and involvement with crime. There may be emotional instability typified by easy laughter or crying, acting drunk, muscular weakness, headaches, impaired equilibrium, and slurred speech.

MERCURY

Mercury compounds are potent neurotoxins. The problem with mercury toxicity is the slow, smoldering effects that never let the person know that mercury is at the root of the problem. Exposure to mercury begins in the womb where the mother transfers mercury to the fetus through the placenta. There are many ways for mercury levels to begin to accumulate. Fetuses are ten times more sensitive to mercury toxicity than adults.

We must have a balance between how much mercury gets into the body and how much we can eliminate. Any organ of the body can be involved, but the most common areas are the brain, liver, and kidneys. Mercury-toxic people are more prone to blushing, loss of self-control, timidity and discouragement. Other symptoms include memory loss, dizziness, anxiety, loss of self confidence, irritability, drowsiness, depression, weight loss, headaches, fatigue, muscle weakness, hearing difficulties, skin inflammation, and being more emotional.

Mercury amalgams (fillings) may be a player in yeast infections and chronic illness. Mercury not only injures tissues and organs, but it is also an antiseptic, attacking microbes in the same way antibiotics do, forcing them to mutate to survive. Microbes learn to defend themselves from such attacks and grow resistant to any treatment that tries to reduce their population.

Common places to find mercury include pesticides, fertilizers, amalgams, drinking water, bleached flour, processed foods, fabric softeners, talc and body powder, mascara, floor waxes and polishes, wood preservatives, plumbing, adhesives, batteries, and air-conditioner filters. Eliminate foods suspected of containing heavy metals, such as swordfish and tuna. The body can accumulate a large quantity of mercury throughout life from many sources.

Mercury is second only to cadmium as being the most toxic heavy metal on the earth. Even exposure to low, yet chronic, levels of mercury can cause problems. Changes in your child's diet and environment, as well as appropriate removal of mercury from the body, are needed.

Chapter 20

ロ

PESTICIDE POISONING

The average child now receives more exposure to pesticides than ever before. In 1993, a landmark study discovered that children are at far greater health risk than was ever realized from the exposure to pesticides in the food supply. The Environmental Protection Agency (EPA) estimates that pesticides contaminate the ground water in at least 38 states. They pollute the drinking water of millions of people. Many of the pesticides that are approved today by the EPA were registered before extensive research was done linking these chemicals to illnesses. The National Coalition Against the Misuse of Pesticides argues that there are no safe pesticides, only acceptable poisons.

Some health-care specialists argue that pesticides make ADD worse in children. Early exposure to these chemicals can cause permanent structural and functional damage to a growing body. They affect the child's immune system, making it harder to fight disease. If a nursing mother has pesticide exposure, she can pass these toxins to her baby.

Organic solvents remain a major problem. It has to be more than coincidental that the present epidemic of hyperactivity and behavioral problems among school children has coincided with steadily increasing levels of volatile organic chemicals found in modern buildings. Behavioral problems may be the earliest sign of chemical toxins. Some common organic solvents are toluene, xylene, acetone, benzene, chloroform, carbon tetrachloride, and trichloroethylene. The potential of these substances for causing brain and neurologic damage is well documented in the medical literature.

COMMON SYMPTOMS OF PESTICIDE POISONING

Toxins absorb easily through the skin and the lungs. The organs most affected are the brain and the nervous system. Common symptoms of pesticide poisoning include the inability to think, impaired memory, poor concentration, poor coordination, and drowsiness. Other symptoms are anxiety, diarrhea, itching and rash, restlessness, headaches, blurred vision, convulsions, pinpoint pupils, dizziness, weakness, nausea, vomiting, muscle pains or twitching, chest pains, disorientation, increased heart rate, loss of feeling, excessive sweating, stomachaches and cramps, increased salivation, breathing difficulties, impaired intellectual functioning and simple motor skills, and irritation of the eyes, throat, and skin.

Organophosphates are now the most widely used pesticides in the United States. These poison the nervous systems of unwanted pests. Children may have continual or repeated exposures to these pesticides through pesticide residues in fruits and vegetables and through their use in or about the school buildings and homes. One study conducted on the effects of pesticides on the nervous system concluded that it is possible that organophosphates may be another cause of brain dysfunction so frequently demonstrated in our younger population.

Most organic solvents and pesticides in use today are fat-soluble and have an affinity for the fatty tissues of the body. The brain and nervous system are more than 25 percent fat in content and are especially vulnerable because of a rich blood supply to these areas. Children and developing fetuses are much more vulnerable to the damaging effects of these toxins because of their rapidly growing tissues and because of the immaturity of their detoxification systems.

Foods contaminated with even low levels of pesticides are known to cause learning and memory impairment, hyperactivity, and aggressive behavior. The possible effects of pesticide residues found in human milk surely deserve investigation. It may be beneficial to test for common pesticides, such as diazinon, because of its common use on crops. Repeated exposure to organophosphate pesticides by children, even at low doses, should cause concern because numerous studies show personality changes and learning disabilities after pesticide exposure. This fact is all the more important when we realize that pesticides may persist in indoor air up to twenty-one days following indoor application and they may persist for months in the fatty tissues of the body. Sadly, the EPA has not yet required testing of pesticides for brain toxicity or to detect neurological defects. Hopefully they will in the near future.

HOW ARE CHILDREN EXPOSED TO PESTICIDES?

The home is the principal place of exposure to pesticides in the United States. Studies show that about 90 percent of all households in this country use pesticides. A wide variety of products are available for home use, including sprays to kill insects on house plants, flea and tick sprays, and shampoos for pets. Other commonly used products are no-pest strips, pesticides to control termites, Kwell shampoo for head lice and scabies, flea collars on pets, pesticides in the garden, and herbicides to control weeds in the yard. Rugs are often moth-proofed, especially if they've ever been put in storage. Rug shampoos may contain insecticides as well. Peelings on fresh fruits and vegetables often contain insecticide and herbicide residues. Tap water can contain these chemicals, too. Insecticides and weed killers can remain in the drinking water if the water-filter unit does not remove these contaminants. All these products increase our body's toxic load.

Insecticides enter the human body through the mouth, lungs, skin, or eyes. Absorption and onset of symptoms by ingestion and inhalation are typically rapid, occurring within a few minutes to a few hours after exposure. Symptoms from skin absorption are generally slower, but can still be dangerous. The body will remove these chemicals in the urine, if possible.

Many third-world countries still use DDT on their foods and then export the food into this country. This country has a ban on DDT, but chemical companies still sell it to Mexico and other countries. With the approval of the General Agreement on Tariffs and Trade (GATT), more pesticide residues will enter this country. Levels of DDT that are much higher than current United States standards will come in on imported peaches and bananas, as well as grapes, strawberries, broccoli, and carrots.

EFFECTS OF PESTICIDE POISONING

The primary target of organophosphate insecticides within the body is an important enzyme required for normal functioning of the nervous system. If enough of this enzyme is inhibited, the nervous system cannot function normally and symptoms may appear. Neurological effects can begin within hours of exposure, or two to three weeks later. They can and do cause behavior and learning deficits that may be irreversible. Even years after the poisoning, persistent symptoms can exist. Nervous system enzymes are present in the blood and can be measured by lab tests. These tests can indicate exposure to organophosphate insecticides.

PESTICIDES IN THE SCHOOL

The biggest offender in the "sick school syndrome" may be pesticides. Most school districts currently manage pests solely by using neurotoxic chemicals, especially organophosphates, in and around schools. The disruption of the central nervous system, with the resultant over stimulation, can lead to hyperactivity, difficulty in focusing attention, impaired verbal ability, difficulty doing math, memory deficits, numbness, tingling, hoarseness, flu-like symptoms, and multiple chemical sensitivities. Less toxic methods of controlling pests need our attention, for the sake of our children.

HOW ARE PESTICIDES TESTED?

When the FDA is determining whether to legalize pesticides, each one is tested in isolation. No one ever tests what happens when a combination of pesticides is used and what effect this might have on the body. Over 500 foods analyzed in a pesticide test had as many as five pesticide residues on them. These combinations have not been tested for toxicity,nor do we have any idea what these mixtures of chemicals are doing to people.

Petroleum-derived chemicals do not occur naturally, so most microorganisms cannot break them down. Pesticides are designed to attack a pest's nervous system, and when humans are exposed to these toxins they can suffer nervous system damage as well. Pesticides contain some of the most toxic synthetic chemicals ever created by humans. The accumulation of such compounds find their way into storage in the fatty parts of each cell. The human body has no previous experience with these chemicals and there is no natural mechanism to break them down, much less eliminate them. The effects may be magnified in the developing nervous systems of children.

A study done in 1993 by the National Academy of Sciences concluded that pesticides posed a significant threat to health. Of course, pesticides are found on our fruits and vegetables, but it is also shocking to learn that most of the pesticides ingested in our country come from animal products. Animals fed pesticide-laden products regularly absorb and store them in their tissues. A large fish will store all the pesticides or toxins stored in the flesh of every one of the smaller fish it has eaten. Each of those smaller fish will collect in its tissues all the pesticides ingested by the even smaller fish they eat. In the same way, farm animals retain in their flesh all the pesticides that they absorb from their feed. Ranchers dip and spray these animals with extremely toxic compounds and feed them massive doses of toxic drugs that are never given to animals raised naturally. Some drugs fed to animals, such as hormones and antibiotics, may also be dangerous for humans.

Whenever you eat the meat or the milk of animals raised with chemicals, you consume concentrated doses of uncontrolled combinations of many of the most deadly chemicals ever known. The EPA reports numerous studies that confirm that animal-origin foods are the major source of pesticide residues in our diet. The desire to reduce the ingestion of toxic chemicals is just one more good reason to reduce your intake of animal products or to buy them chemical and pesticide-free.

As our food supply becomes more contaminated with pesticides, we need to make greater demands for healthy foods in the marketplace. If consumers begin to look for and demand safer food, farmers will be forced to reduce their use of pesticides and make changes that will significantly benefit our health and protect the environment. Write your congressional representatives, the FDA and the EPA. Alert them to your concerns. Methods to produce food with little or no pesticides have existed for many years and the nation's food producers must be encouraged to switch to these methods. Through your choices in the supermarket, you can send a direct message to the food industry.

Commercial farming techniques have stripped our soils of vital trace minerals, and left residues of dangerous chemicals in our fruits and vegetables, as well as in our meats. Your body is a by-product of the soil that grows your food. It can only be as healthful as the source. Remember, pesticides are poison. Their use is profit-based, not health-based. Our bodies were never intended to be exposed to toxic chemicals. Chemical insecticides and pesticides are producing ailments that physicians cannot even identify—ailments like ADD.

Section Four

WHAT ELSE?

OTHER POSSIBLE CAUSES OF ADD

Chapter 21

THE
UNDERACTIVE
THYROID

L
ocated just below the Adam's apple is a tiny butterfly-shaped gland called the thyroid. Weighing less than an ounce, this gland has an enormous effect on your health. It controls all aspects of the body's metabolism—the rate at which tissues use fats and carbohydrates, and the maintenance of body temperature. The thyroid also helps regulate the production of protein and controls the heart beat rate. To maintain the ideal metabolism, your thyroid must constantly release the correct amount of hormones. The hypothalamus and pituitary glands control the rate that hormones are released from the thyroid. These hormones are essential for keeping the brain at a high energy level all the time.

Hyperthyroidism is a condition causing the thyroid to release an excessive amount of hormones. This can speed up your metabolism as much as 60 to 80 percent. Hypothyroidism is a more likely condition, when the hormone levels your thyroid releases are too low. An underactive thyroid, both prenatal and during childhood, severely limits development of the brain.

Sometimes the symptoms of thyroid problems are so subtle that the condition goes undiagnosed. Thyroid function tests have improved over the last twenty years, but they sometimes fail to detect mild cases of hypothyroidism. I have found a lab test to be normal on several occasions, but the children in question still had many symptoms indicating a thyroid dysfunction. An imbalance in thyroid hormone can have an effect on energy and behavior. It seems that hypothyroid children, in an effort to fight fatigue resulting from low thyroid function, will stay in constant motion. Some children with a mild condition are lethargic, but if your child seems hyperactive don't assume that she has too much rather than too little thyroid activity. One boy I know was so hyperactive and restless that he was placed in a special school. He also lacked normal muscular coordination, a characteristic of many children with a low-functioning thyroid. Thyroid therapy improved his symptoms. The following year, he attended regular school and is now a quiet, studious student who keeps up academically with his classmates.

HOW ARE HYPOTHYROIDISM AND ADD RELATED?

Other symptoms of an underactive thyroid include sluggishness, cold hands or feet, constipation, a puffy face, hoarse voice, and pale, dry skin. Some people gain weight and retain fluids. Forgetfulness and slowing of the thought processes can develop. There may be a short attention span and limited ability to concentrate. Other symptoms may be irritability, slow reaction time, depression, a tendency to be quarrelsome, as well as a lack of cooperation. As the condition progresses, symptoms become more noticeable. Constant over-stimulation of the thyroid to release more hormones can lead to a goiter (enlarged thyroid). Sometimes the only definite physical finding in the child is fatigue or a subnormal basal body temperature.

Hypothyroidism in childhood severely limits development of the brain and may be an important component of hyperactivity and ADD. The brain and nerve cells need thyroid hormone (along with its co-factor magnesium) to produce enough energy to become quietly relaxed. For years, some physicians have known of the quieting effects of thyroid hormone, prescribing it for hyperactive children.

Since 1950, the increase in the incidence of hyperactivity in children has steadily gone up. One of the reasons is the increased use of unsaturated vegetable oils. Unsaturated oils can interfere with thyroid secretion, the transport of thyroid hormone in the blood, and the response of the tissue thyroid receptors. Other possible causes of thyroid dysfunction could be autoimmune disorder, thyroid surgery, or treatment with radioactive iodine to treat an excessively active thyroid resulting in the gland becoming underactive. A low thyroid could also be the result of a pituitary disorder. Approximately 1 in 5,000 newborns have a defective thyroid gland or no gland at all.

In the early 1900s, hypothyroidism and the development of goiter were common in the midwest and Great Lakes regions of the United States. Iodine was lacking in the water and soil of these areas. Without enough dietary iodine, the thyroid cannot make iodine-containing hormones. After scientists recognized iodine deficiency as one of the causes of hypothyroidism, iodized salt was introduced. Since then, surgery to remove large goiters is rarely necessary. Even if you don't use iodized table salt, most people get enough iodine because of the addition of iodized salt to many processed foods. Iodine naturally occurs in water, dairy products, and seafood.

A child's symptoms, along with the results of a blood test, usually determine the diagnosis of an underactive thyroid. Using the results of thyroid tests, a large study screened for thyroid abnormalities in 277 children with ADD. They concluded that the amount of thyroid abnormalities was higher (5.4 percent) in children with ADD than in the normal population (less than 1 percent).

An old and useful test of thyroid function uses the Achilles tendon reflex to observe the relaxation speed of the calf muscle. In hypothyroid states, the muscle is slow to relax because the cells are slow to replace the energy used. The muscles tend to fatigue easily and to swell and feel sore with moderate exercise. In children, these painful, swollen, and tense muscles sometimes make it hard to go to sleep after an active day.

If your child's symptoms are caused by an under- or overactive thyroid, then it is best to treat the problem, rather than just trying to control the symptoms. Traditional medicine usually treats this condition with hormone replacement drugs. This medication is usually lifelong. There are several natural treatments available to restore the thyroid back to normal in a shorter time. Sometimes, it takes only a few days of treatment to feel better. Sometimes the treatment for a thryroid condition involves just dietary changes, but more often there is a need for a thyroid supplement. Try a natural thyroid product first before using hormone replacement therapy.

Chapter 22

⎁

SEEING, HEARING, FEELING—THE SENSES AND ADD

When making sure their child is healthy enough to enter school, many parents overlook a very important thing—vision. Most people think that if a child's vision is 20/20 then everything is fine. What needs to be understood is that vision is more than just clarity. It also includes binocular coordination, speed accomodation, vertical movement and other visual functions necessary to visualize, understand, and apply the information that comes through the eyes. Children with 20/20 sight may not have these abilities, and this results in learning problems. Difficulties arise because vision impaired children rarely report symptoms. They think everyone sees the same as they do. A typical school or a doctor's office doesn't help the situation because they usually only identify children who cannot see clearly. Functions such as binocular coordination and speed of accommodation are not measured at all.

Our two eyes are supposed to work together—to perform as one entity. This is a skill that must be acquired through use during the preschool years. Not all children adequately develop visual skill and this can interfere with comprehension, the ability to perceive spatial relations, and the ability to concentrate. For example, there may be visual discomfort or distortions of the text while reading. This reduces close attention to details and sustained mental effort. As a result, a child will be easily distracted. The signs of inattention are not only observable, but also many times interpreted (or misinterpreted) simply as ADD. Reducing or eliminating the visual disorder can lead to significant improvement in attention status.

Another kind of visual-motor problem controls the ability to focus both eyes on the same object at the same time. Without this function, our brain receives two different pictures at the same time. The eyes do not work together smoothly as an object moves closer. We know this as double vision. The eyes may also have poor staying power as they read. This results in distractibility, eye strain, tiredness, headaches, and poor comprehension. These deficits lead to poor eye-hand coordination, clumsiness, performance problems and again, the misdiagnosis of ADD-hyperactivity.

Yet another visual problem is the inability to control the horizontal or vertical eye movement required to track words across, or up and down a page. The problem is not vision, but a lack of motor control. Children with this problem find reading very stressful. Some are unable to perceive the detailed form of letters. Vision therapy corrects these problems through training. It teaches the child to control their eyes so that they can make rapid and accurate discrimination between similar letters, such as "b" and "d." Without correction these children may appear disinterested. Most children with reading disabilities have measurable and correctable problems. If these problems are allowed to continue, then their adult life can result in needless suffering with headaches and confusion stemming from poor visual processing.

Vision therapy is the generally accepted treatment for various developmental visual disorders that may effect attentiveness, social and school performance. Vision training is not necessarily a cure for ADD, or an immediate substitute for necessary medications, but rather a component of treatment.

SYMPTOMS OF VISION PROBLEMS

Remember that school is not the only place where it is important to learn, read, and focus. The following list of symptoms can often accompany vision problems:

• Gets drowsy in class
• Avoids reading
• Headaches or nausea after reading
• Double vision or print blurs
• Reddened eyes or lids; encrusted eyelids; frequent sties on eyelids
• Burning or itching eyes
• Eye strain, rubs eyes, blinks often
• Complains about bright lights
• Has poor comprehension or loses place when reading; uses finger to keep place
• Omits or substitutes words; skips lines when reading
• Writes uphill or downhill; writing is poorly spaced or crooked; unable to stay on ruled lines
• Poor blackboard-to-desk copying
• Fails to complete work on time and/or takes a very long time to complete homework
• Holds book very close, tilts head, covers one eye, moves head while reading
• Poor attentive skills
• Misjudges size and distance
• Has slow reaction time in sports or play

Find an optometrist that works with children who have perceptual and visual problems and specializes in problems such as tracking movement, building balance, spatial relationships, and coordination. Optometric vision therapy is an individualized program directed at treatment of specifically diagnosed vision conditions. The use of lenses, prisms and specialized testing and training procedures are part of the successful treatment. Among school-age children, vision disorders affect one in every four. Early intervention is very important. Once a child enters school, the pattern of academic and social failures begin.

As an example of positive change, I include the history of a child that did go to a behavioral optometrist. This boy was found to have a problem tracking, focusing, and teaming his eyes together. The lack of coordination with his eyes was causing double vision, and this caused much of his attention and concentration problems. Lenses were prescribed along with a behavioral program. This immediately helped improve the visual motor system. Within three weeks the double vision disappeared. After six months of vision therapy, this child scored twenty points higher on IQ tests than he had previously. His behavior and learning improved and his task completion and organization also improved. He received better grades and began working up to his potential. He was no longer a disruptive child in the classroom.

If your child exhibits any of the symptoms listed in this chapter, a comprehensive learning-related vision exam will need to be done. This will test the need for glasses, as well as other visual problems. For more information on finding a behavioral optometrist in your area, consult the "Resource Guide" at the end of this book.

SCREENING A CHILD'S HEARING

Even when a child hears perfectly well, parents will notice times when their child doesn't seem to listen, when the child simply tunes out. But what if a child doesn't hear well? What if he tries to listen, but is incapable of distinguishing sounds? Until there is a detectable problem with a child's speech and understanding, chances are that no one will realize he has a hearing problem. If this goes undetected until the age of 24 to 30 months, it is likely to cause impaired language development that leads to problems with learning and academic success.

Obviously, it is necessary to identify a child with a hearing problem as soon as possible. This increases chances of the child's normal development. Maybe there should be hearing tests for all infants.

Hearing screening for infants in the United States has been available for a long time, but it has been time-consuming and expensive. Usually, doctors only test high-risk infants. These are premature babies with low birth weight who have been in intensive care. They may have a family history of deafness. Unfortunately, about half of the children who end up with permanent hearing loss are not in these high-risk categories. By the time anyone notices a hearing problem, language problems are already present.

Today there is a new screening test available that is simple and economical. It is the Otoacoustic Emissions Test (OAE) developed by British physicist David Kemp. When the ear is working correctly, it will echo a series of clicks sounded in the ear canal. After placing a small device resembling an ear plug into the infant's ear, the computer monitor displays the results as a jagged bright blue section on a graph. Then an audiologist interprets them. The test only takes from 15 seconds to two minutes for each ear.

Infants should have their hearing tested shortly after birth. If they fail the first test, the test should be repeated at two weeks of age. Around eight percent of babies screened exhibit a hearing loss with the first test, but eighty-five percent of these babies go on to pass the second test. If there is permanent hearing loss, children as young as three months can be fitted with hearing aids. They will not miss out on proper language development that could influence how well they learn in the future.

Much of the information in a classroom is presented to children verbally. It is very difficult for a child experiencing auditory processing problems to gain information when the teacher speaks while writing on the blackboard. This means the teacher's back is to the students, and the child is unable to read the teacher's face. Parents have often told me that they must speak to the child face to face to be understood. If your child frequently does not seem to hear you, consider having them tested for hearing loss.

Children with repeated cases of ear infections are more likely to end up with hearing loss. This can impair speech and language development, lower general intelligence scores and create learning difficulties. Ear infections are twice as common in learning-disabled children as non-learning-disabled children. Preventive treatment is important since many of the factors associated with hyperactivity are also associated with ear infections. In one study, there was an association between recurrent ear infection in infancy and later hyperactivity. Almost 70 percent of the children being evaluated for school failure, who were also receiving medication for hyperactivity, gave a history of more than ten ear infections. Children with recurrent ear infections receive repeated and prolonged courses of broad-spectrum antibiotic drugs. These drugs cause alterations in gut flora including the proliferation of *Candida albicans*. Bowel changes promote the absorption of food antigens and put the child at risk for food allergies. This may play a major role in causing hyperactivity, attention deficit syndrome, and related behavior and learning problems.

TOUCH AND MOVEMENT

I often wonder whatever happened to the cradle. It used to be a common practice to keep a baby in a cradle, a cradle that was near the center of the mother's home-making activities by day and moved next to the parents' bed at night. In the cradle the baby could be rocked to sleep with regularity. Today's infants, on the other hand, go from the stationary bassinet to an immobile crib. Yet for nine months the child in the womb was carried and rocked gently as the mother went about her day. Then, abruptly after birth, the child experiences long stretches of stillness and silence; being touched and moved around is often limited to feedings and bath time. When the baby is carried anywhere, it is often in a plastic carrier which doesn't even give direct contact with the warmth of the parent's arms.

The reason a discussion of movement and touch is necessary is because their importance is just now beginning to be recognized by the scientific community. Recent studies analyzed the role that movement plays in normal child development. It was found that the absence of movement, along with the absence of touching and cuddling, can lead to learning and behavior disorders in children. Receiving enough loving and physical contact throughout childhood—beginning in infancy—can affect a child throughout life.

In many "primitive" cultures, mothers carry babies on their chest, hip, or back. They hold them in a wrap-around cloth, sling, or papoose-type frame, or some similar device. When they are not carried, they place the infant in a small hammock near the mother's working area. The child is always within sight, and the mother talks to them and rocks them frequently. In the country of Bali, for example, the mother carries the baby in her arms for the first few months of life, then in a hip sling until about the child is two years of age. The baby is rarely out of someone's arms except during the daily bath. All waking and sleeping activities take place within this physical bond of being held and touched by the mother and other family members. Interestingly, the Balinese are one of the most nonviolent cultures, noted for an almost complete absence of violence and hostility in adults.

In a cross-cultural study of 49 cultures, there was a clear correlation between the lack of physical affection, particularly touching and movement in the early years, and a high degree of adult crimes. The National Institute of Child Health says abnormal social and emotional behaviors that occur later in life result from early deprivation of touching, contact, and movement. These abnormalities include depression, autistic behavior, and hyperactivity in the younger years. We can promote happier children by paying greater attention to the infant's need to touch and move.

A beneficial stimulation occurs in the equilibrium center of the brain when a baby is in motion. This stimulates the brain cells and regulates other important brain functions that control normal physical, mental, psychological and social development. A lack of sensory impulses to this brain center may be responsible for learning difficulties. Another problem is poor sensory integration. Being ready to learn reading, writing, and arithmetic is related to good sensory-motor integration. This results partly from plenty of touching and movement in infancy and early childhood.

One of the midbrain's function is to filter incoming stimuli that the brain receives. It also prioritizes the incoming messages and directs them to the appropriate location in the brain. When this part of the brain is not functioning properly the child may be unable to devote attention to one subject at a time. It is a frequent suggestion that students with ADD and memory problems be given memory exercises, or be asked to carry a notebook. These students are told to focus and concentrate. The problem may not be a deficit of attention, but an overabundance of it. These students cannot focus on one thing because they are unable to filter out peripheral stimuli or prioritize information. They simply cannot decide what they should do first. Background activity, such as rustling papers, cars passing, and other people's conversations, all receive the same amount of attention as the desired activity.

The development of the neuropathways in the brain increases as children grow. If children do not have the opportunity to do activities that correspond with each stage of development, then they will not reach their neurological potential. Examples of these necessary activities are using both eyes at the same time, recognizing and distinguishing symbols, understanding words, touching things, crawling, creeping, walking upright, running, swinging arms, skipping, other activities that require coordination and balance, communicating with speech, and picking up and manipulating small objects.

Sensory input and motor activities develop the proper sequence of neurological functioning and are essential for the development of learning. Learning is a sensory process that must be reinforced by motor functioning. If input is nonexistent, limited, or confused, the sensory pathways will not develop correctly. The person has to begin again with activities and sensory inputs that have proven beneficial in promoting effective neurological organization from early infancy on. This means that it is necessary to retrace steps in the normal process of developing going back as far as possible. Children with ADD may benefit by the same sensory and motor activities as assigned in the program prescribed by a neurodevelopmental therapist. They base these programs on increased stimulation in six sensory and motor areas: visual, auditory, touching, mobility, language, and manual skills.

Children who have not reached the peak of their neurological development find it difficult to do the required classroom work. Children with immature nervous systems often seem to be misbehaving, or not making an effort. They may not have the capacity to meet these challenges yet. If you have a child with learning or behavior problems, and you believe your child did not get adequate physical holding and movement in their development, look into sensory integration therapy. See the "Resource Guide" for more information.

Chapter 23

MISCELLANEOUS FACTORS

Throughout this book, various explanations of ADD-like behavior have been explored. While the major possible causes have already been discussed, there are still a few other possibilities that warrant our attention.

ASTHMATIC CHILDREN TAKING THEOPHYLLINE

At least three studies of asthmatic children show a relationship between learning and behavioral problems and the use of theophylline. This is a common medication used for asthmatics. When the children took approximately ten to twenty micrograms, adverse effects in school behavior and performance resulted.

BLOOD PRESSURE

One of the functions of the autonomic nervous system is to raise blood pressure. If your child has chronic low blood pressure, then she is unable to circulate enough blood and oxygen to the brain to stay alert. The hyperactivity may be a way for the body to raise the blood pressure to a level that is sufficient to insure circulation to the brain. This may be one reason why hyperactivity can be reduced by taking Ritalin. Ritalin is a stimulant and raises blood pressure.

If your child does have low blood pressure, then requiring him to sit still for a period of time is not helpful. Asking your child to run around the block or do some jumping jacks will raise the blood pressure and enable him to be alert and more quiet for a period of time.

BRAIN INJURIES

Over the last decades, scientists have come up with many possible theories about what causes ADD. Some of these theories have led to dead ends, while others have led to exciting new avenues of investigation. One disappointing theory was that all attention disorders and learning disabilities were caused by minor head injuries or undetectable damage to the brain. It was thought that ADD resulted from an early infection or complications at birth. Because of this theory, these disorders were called "minimal brain damage" or "minimal brain dysfunction." Certain types of head injury can explain some cases of attention disorder, but not everyone with ADD or a learning disability has a history of head trauma or birth complications.

BRAIN CONNECTIONS

Researchers are looking for all types of differences between those who do and those who do not have ADD. Finding out how the brain normally develops in the fetus offers some clues about what may disrupt the process. Brain imaging studies using PET scanners (Positron Emission Tomography) has shown that brain metabolism is lower in children with ADD. More important, these studies show significantly lower metabolic activity in regions of the brain that control attention, social judgment, and movement. This may demonstrate a link between a person's ability to pay continued attention and the level of activity in the brain.

Biochemical studies have documented that some children with ADD have lower levels of a number of neurotransmitters, including dopamine. Successful medications for these children affect the levels of several neurotransmitters in the brain.

DEVELOPMENTAL DELAY

Developmentally delayed children account for one type of ADD with hyperactivity. These children are unable to control their behavior because their control center does not develop as rapidly as does the motor division of the body. Sending these children to school when they are older may be a better choice for them. This allows time for fine muscle coordination to develop. Boys suffer from learning disabilities more frequently than girls because their development is slower than girls until puberty. Then they usually catch up and the level of activity decreases. Concentration and attention span also improve.

DRUG USE

Scientists at the National Institutes of Health and other research institutions are tracking clues to determine what might prevent nerve cells from forming the proper connections. Some of the factors they are studying include drug use during pregnancy, toxins, and genetics. Research shows that a mother's use of cigarettes, alcohol, or other drugs during pregnancy may have damaging effects on the unborn child. These substances may be dangerous to the developing brain of the fetus and distort developing nerve cells.

There is a known link between heavy alcohol use during pregnancy and fetal alcohol syndrome (FAS), a condition that can lead to low birth weight, intellectual impairment, and certain physical defects. Many children born with FAS show the same hyperactivity, inattention, and impulsivity as children with ADD. Drugs such as cocaine, including the smokable form known as crack, seem to affect the normal development of brain receptors. These brain cells help to transmit incoming signals from our skin, eyes, and ears, and helps control our responses to the environment. Drug abuse may harm these receptors. Some scientists believe that such damage may lead to ADD.

FAMILY HISTORY

It is becoming more evident that hyperactive parents have children with the same problem. This history is so common that it suggests the strong possibility of genetically determined ADD. Children with ADD usually have at least one close relative with ADD. At least one-third of all fathers who had ADD in their youth bear children who have ADD. It is even more convincing that the majority of identical twins share the trait. At NIH researchers are also on the trail of a gene that may be involved in transmitting ADD in a small number of families with a genetic thyroid disorder. There may also be a correlation between hyperactive children who are very sugar sensitive and who have a family history of alcoholism, sugar cravings, or diabetes.

Fate may have handed your child some negative genetic traits, but many of them can be offset. Genes determine susceptibility to certain diseases, but many conditions or diseases don't have to manifest, unless your lifestyle and diet allow them to surface. Making diet or lifestyle changes could keep your particular family disease from appearing or could minimize its effects.

OVER-STIMULATION

Over-stimulation from television and competitive games may lead to hyperactivity. The constant and rapid change of visual images seen on television and their violent content may cause a stimulating effect on sensitive children. With the frequent change of scenes the attention span is trained to be short. Children with overly taxed nervous systems often indulge in unfocused activity.

Television can further the adverse effects of ADD. Children spend more time in front of the TV than they are spending in school, playing outdoors, or reading. Some of the adverse effects of TV are that it promotes and encourages snacking on junk foods, decreases outdoor activity, increases electromagnetic radiation, encourages aggressive behavior and interferes with studies. It also promotes poor social skills since the child does not spend time interacting with other children. It encourages weight gain because of the lack of exercise and eating a poor diet.

PARASITES

Some children with severe behavioral problems and hyperactivity are also diagnosed with parasites. I know of one child diagnosed with ADD who later was found to have a parasite-caused infection called schistosomiasis. This is a common parasite in Egypt, where it is found in freshwater snails who serve as the parasite's intermediate host. This child had not been to Egypt, but had played with snails in his backyard. He then undoubtedly put his unwashed hands in his mouth. After the proper treatment to rid him of schistosomiasis, the child's hyperactivity diminished and his behavior became normal.

SMOKING

Childhood exposure to maternal smoking can result in low birth weights, infant mortality, respiratory infection, asthma, and modest impairment of cognitive function. A 1992 study presented in *Pediatrics* evaluated maternal smoking and behavior problems among 2,256 children, ages four through eleven. The children's behavior problems increased with exposure to maternal cigarette smoke. A child is three times more likely to be hyperactive if the mother smokes 23 or more cigarettes a day during pregnancy than if she does not smoke at all. This may be because the decrease in blood flow to the placenta that occurs in smokers retards the development of the fetus.

STRESS

Some children's hyperactive states improve when someone focuses their attention. They then become quiet and interested in what is going on. They need an additional stress factor to trigger their hyperactive state. Some children are very hyperactive at school, but appear "normal" at home. This may indicate that the nature of the stress is variable or appears only at school.

VACCINATIONS

It has been noted that there is an increase in behavior difficulties such as hyperactivity, attention deficit, and learning disabilities in children after receiving vaccinations. There is a known interaction between the nervous and immune system, and injuries to one system affect the other. Stories abound of parents who observe changes in the personality of their children following their immunizations. Some children are just never the same. These observations by parents deserve some notice by the medical community.

Archie Kalokerinos, an Australian medical doctor, wrote a book some years ago called *Every Second Child.* He writes about the deaths among aborigine children after government doctors gave these children their DTP immunization shots. He found that about 50 percent of the children who received vaccinations died. Archie knew it was the shots. The impoverished diet of these people did nothing to support the immune system. Without adequate vitamins and minerals available, the stress of the shots wiped them out. To counteract the effects of the shots, he personally supplied each child in his district with the appropriate amount of vitamin C. Not another child died. Archie is convinced that the DTP shots are the most likely cause of Sudden Infant Death Syndrome. What if the DTP shot causes other problems beside the sudden death of infants?

Section Five

TREATING

ADD

Chapter 24

The New Biofeedback

Neurotherapy, a form of biofeedback, is a relatively new approach to ADD. It began in the mid 1970s, but there were few well-controlled clinical research studies until recently. The few that were published, however, were impressive. A study by Joel Lubar, Ph.D., focused on therapy that decreased theta brain waves. Lower theta wave frequency reduced or eliminated ADD symptoms. Training that increased theta brain waves brought the symptoms back. Michael Tansey, Ph.D., has published small but similarly impressive studies for over fifteen years.

Recently, there has been an increase number of reports published on the effectiveness of neurotherapy. Two new organizations have formed to provide a professional forum for discussion, presentation of papers, and teaching. These are the Society for the Study of Neuronal Regulation and the EEG Section of the Association for Applied Psychophysiology and Biofeedback. The latter organization has been in existence for twenty-five years, focusing on biofeedback research and practice. There is a certifying board, the National Registry of Neurofeedback Providers, that certifies care providers in the practice of neurotherapy.

It has been possible to reduce seizures using biofeedback since 1960. Training to reduce slow-waves and increase certain other brain waves were very helpful in reducing seizures in both animals and humans. By displaying the differences in brain waves, these machines help train people to alter their own brain waves. Now one of the approaches to treating ADD is the use of an electroencephalogram (EEG). An EEG is a graphic record of the electrical activity of the brain as recorded by a machine called an electroencephalograph. Children can sometimes be helped with this device to control and modify their behavior.

Biofeedback is a training program designed to teach a child to control involuntary or unfelt events, such as their own activity level and concentration. During an EEG biofeedback session, sensors from a machine are placed on the child's head. Brain waves are displayed on a video screen in an interactive "game" format. A sophisticated computer program teaches the child to change brain waves in order to score "points" on the game. The computer is set to make sounds and change screen displays that act as "feedback."

Feedback makes learned self-control possible since it teaches the child how to change his or her performance based on feedback about that performance. Just like learning any new skill, it takes practice and time. On average a child needs between 20 to 40 sessions before the learned behavior can be applied without conscious effort.

Numerous studies show distinctly identifiable EEG abnormalities in children with ADD, learning disabilities, and hyperactivity. The majority of these children have an increase in slow-wave activity and a decrease in fast-wave activity. This becomes more evident when a child is performing academic tasks. Slow-wave activity is associated with wandering thoughts or daydreaming. Fast-wave activity is associated with concentration, attention, and an alert, waking consciousness. Teaching these children to be aware of and increase their "fast" brain waves, and inhibit the "slow" brain waves, gives them more control over their undesirable behavior.

One must see the brainwaves of people with ADD, with or without hyperactivity, to understand that it may be a disorder of relative "under-arousal." When stimulated, children with ADD display smaller and/or slower than normal brain reactions to stimuli. More "sleepy" or low-frequency patterns appear in the brain's electrical activity. This excessively slow wave activity is often most pronounced during reading or listening tasks. The brain activity can look much like stage-two sleep while the person is trying to read. ADD is marked by an increase in "sleepy waves" in the EEG.

This may be why amphetamine-type medications work on children with ADD. What seems to happen is that the children's brains are getting stimulated enough by the drug to allow them to focus and pay attention. The hyperactivity may be a coping mechanism to maintain something like normal arousal. When a hyperactive child first learns to sit still, they rapidly drop off into a drowsy state, seeming to live at the edge of sleep.

Neurofeedback lets a child instantly know when he is slightly more attentive, more focused and less sleepy. The increase in alertness is initially small and momentary. A great deal of coaching and reinforcement needs to be done during the training sessions as the child practices with the computer display. The computer produces tones so the child can tell when he is paying better attention during reading, listening, doing math, conversing, and other school/work tasks.

The therapy part of neurotherapy involves several things. A therapist establishes a strong rapport with the child and skillfully encourages new levels of effort. Also crucial is the imparting of study skills, good attitudes, and self esteem, along with assertiveness training and listening skills. Using biofeedback in conjunction with other techniques appears to have promise for reducing some of the behavioral symptoms of ADD. Behavioral intervention does not eliminate the problem, but can make a chronic condition manageable. Neurofeedback does not wear off and does not rely on drugs to change behavior. It improves the symptoms of distractibility, hyperactivity, impulsivity, and even learning disabilities. Specific reports of improvement in symptoms include:

- becoming calmer
- being more focused
- being more thoughtful
- measured intelligence increased between 12 and 20 points
- reducing or eliminating medication
- improvement of dyslexia and other learning disabilities
- being less oppositional
- fewer night terrors
- improved self-esteem
- less frustration
- improved handwriting ability
- fewer headaches
- becoming more playful
- having a better sense of humor

Unlike many forms of therapy in clinical settings, EEG biofeedback integrates training to real-world environments. It does this in four ways:

1) by performing actual school tasks with school books during the neurofeedback session
2) by coaching the parents to notice and reward increases in alertness, improvements in memory, improvements in follow-through, improvements in impulse control, etc.
3) by coaching the child to notice changes in alertness and attention states with the aim of enhancing voluntary alertness as the child becomes more skillful
4) by working with the family to help them turn what is often an upsetting situation into a cooperative adventure in coaching, tolerance, ups and downs, frustration, communication, and joy

This type of treatment takes an investment in time, effort, and money. The course of treatment with neurotherapy is about three to five months, depending on scheduling. The typical treatment takes between twenty and forty sessions and sometimes more in complicated cases. The cost can range between $1500 and $3000 with insurance sometimes covering the expense. The cost of evaluating ADD and providing individual and family counseling is usually covered by insurance. Ask for references from both people who have had successful treatments, and from those who have not found benefit from using biofeedback.

When I ask children who have used biofeedback what has changed the most for them, the usual reply is "I can pay attention all the way through class now." Biofeedback is not a "cure" for ADD, nor a substitute for any necessary medication, but one more component of treatment that may allow your child to learn more effectively.

A recent study looked at eighteen males age ten to thirteen years old who were diagnosed as hyperactive. Six received biofeedback, six took ten to fifteen milligrams of Ritalin a day, and six regularly played a game with the research assistant. Validity was determined by pre and post-treatment scores on the most accepted rating scales (Conner's Teacher Rating Scale, the Werry-Weiss-Peter's Scale, and the Zukow Parent Rating Scale). Only the biofeedback group significantly improved.

Biofeedback is closely aligned to changing the basic functioning of a child. Though not all family situations lend themselves to trying biofeedback and behavioral modification, excellent results still are frequently seen, especially when patients are willing. If you are frustrated by your child's progress in school or behavior at home, you should consider EEG biofeedback as a possible adjunct to treatment. If your child has a learning disability that has not responded well to individualized instruction or additional tutoring, then EEG biofeedback is certainly worth a try.

Chapter 25

⎡⎦

HOMEOPATHY, CELL SALTS AND FLOWER ESSENCES

H omeopathy is a therapeutic system of medicine developed by Samuel Hahnemann nearly 200 years ago in Germany. It is now accepted as a way to treat a wide range of physical and emotional problems in just about every country in the world. Homeopathy is based upon the "law of similars" or "like cures like." This means that a substance administered in large crude dosages to a healthy individual will produce specific symptoms, but when this material has been reduced in size and administered in minute doses, it will stimulate the body's reactive process to relieve these symptoms. Ipecac is a good example. If this substance is taken in large quantities it produces vomiting, but taken in minute doses it can cure vomiting.

Homeopathic medications can be used effectively for many conditions and illnesses, including ADD. These medications are completely safe and non-addictive even for babies and small children. In the majority of conditions, the response to treatment compares favorably with conventional methods, but there are none of the often disastrous side effects of the typical conventional prescriptions. When there is an underlying emotional factor, homeopathic results are often superior. Children maintain their improvement and are not dependent upon their pills once they make an initial improvement.

Homeopathy is concerned with the treatment of the whole person rather than treating the disease alone. For this reason, people with the same condition may often be treated with different homeopathic remedies. Homeopathy is a healing process that stimulates and encourages the body's natural healing forces of recovery. Conventional medicine believes that symptoms are caused by the illness, but homeopathy sees the symptoms as the body's natural reaction in fighting the illness and seeks to stimulate rather than suppress these symptoms.

The homeopathic treatment of ADD in children is based on a very careful history of the child's behavior. This can be told by the child, as well as the parents and teachers. For those who have been raised on orthodox medicine and prescription drugs, the use of homeopathic medication seems like an impossible fantasy. It usually takes a high potency of the appropriate homeopathic remedy to get results, but this may not be available over-the-counter from health food stores. I suggest that you consult with someone trained in homeopathy. Some remedies only represent a thin layer of symptoms that need to be removed before the real remedy is revealed. A subsequent homeopathic remedy may be needed. Each remedy below has a set of symptoms that it treats best. See if one of them fits your child.

There are more than 2,000 homeopathic remedies containing very small quantities of the substances called potencies. They may look the same as other medicines, but they are totally different in their preparation and action. They are usually presented in the form of granules, tables, or liquids. Homeopathic remedies are prepared in modern labs with the highest quality standards and derived from pure, natural animal, vegetable, or mineral substances that are listed in the *Homeopathic Pharmacopoeia of the United States.*

The granules should be allowed to dissolved in the mouth or under the tongue, preferable free from strongly flavored substances.

The prescribed number of drops should be placed under the tongue and held there for about a minute. These medicines are best taken apart from food or drink, about 15 minutes. Avoid handling to prevent contamination. Keep the medicines in a cool, dark place away from strong-smelling substances and they will remain effective for several years. Do not expose your child to strong odors such as Lysol, fresh paint, or eucalyptus used in steam baths. Strong odors will antidote the homeopathic remedies. Never expose the medicines to direct sunlight, electric blankets, caffeine, mint, raw garlic, X-rays, or cigarette smoke (especially menthol).

If you are experienced with the use of homeopathy, then the following list of remedies may be helpful in determining which one best suites your child. This section is not meant to be a course on homeopathy, cell salts, or flower essences. You may need to read further on these types of natural medications or seek professional help.

ANACARDIUM

The anacardium remedy is used for children who express bizarre features and convictions, including the feeling of being followed or having a double. These children feel as if they have two wills, each commanding or moving them to do opposite things, or one commanding them to do something while the other commands them not to do it. Mentally, they seem confused with a tendency to curse and swear. Anacardium children are abusive to animals and often defiant and malicious to people. Low self-esteem predominates. There are complaints of a sensation that feels like a band around the body or that the bowels feel blocked by a plug with constipation often present.

ARSENICUM ALBUM

This remedy is used for children who are extremely hyperactive and have allergies. They tend to feel cold and overdress on the warmest summer day. Because of their constant fidgety movements and activity, they are often exhausted, weak, and unable to think clearly. Sleep is restless with much tossing and turning. Their mind is never at rest because of obsessional thinking and double-checking. Agitation is predominant, varying from agitated anxiety to agitated states of depression. Time passes too slowly for them and they are always in a hurry and exasperated. Their face may not reveal any true expression of joy, relaxation, or contentment. These children are inflexible with a tendency to deny problems. They need company and people because they fear being left alone. Arsenicum children worry about the past rather than the future.

BARYTA CARBONICA

This remedy may be useful for the child that shows extreme delay in mental and physical development. The appetite may be voracious, but they still grow poorly because of defective assimilation. There may be emaciation of the rest of the body, while the abdomen is greatly enlarged. These children have difficulty keeping up with mental tasks. They are shy with a lack of understanding of the world, taking things literally, acting silly to cover-up inadequacies, but acting violent and having school phobia. The child suffers from changes in the weather, especially when it is damp and cold. Inflamed, swollen and suppurated tonsils are a consequence of the least exposure to cold that may also result in a chronic cough.

CANNABIS INDICA

Cannabis is used for children who are "spaced out" and autistic. They love things of the senses. All perceptions, sensations, and emotions are exaggerated to the utmost degree. Ecstasy may alternate rapidly with depression. Distances seem infinite and time endless. Surroundings are distorted and colors have increased brilliance. They make up stories and act to cover them up. Some mental disturbances include absent-mindedness, short attention span, daydreaming, fixed ideas, fear of death, and biting themselves or others. These children can not stand heat in any form and feel faint in a hot stuffy room. Their appetite is often ravenous with excessive thirst for cold water, along with a fear of drinking. Drowsiness is prominent and sleep tends to be noisy and accompanied by teeth grinding. The child wakes suddenly jerking the limbs. Urinary tract problems are common.

CAPSICUM

These children are homesick, discontented, brooding, irritable, absent-minded, disobedient, and angry. They seem obstinate in the extreme. This child may want something, but will oppose it if suggested by someone else. Capsicum children fear being censured and are offended easily. They are restless, clumsy, and run into everything. It is hard for them to sleep at night, but yawn during the day. They wake in a fright, screaming, or full of fear. The least air draft makes them worse, even if the air is warm.

CARCINOSIN

These children appear dull of mind, disinterested, and have an aversion to conversation. They are fearful, timid, unhappy, worried, and obstinate, yet sensitive to reprimand and music. They are often sympathetic to others. This child may be very tidy or the opposite. They love to travel and will over-extend themselves. There may be a brownish cafe-au-lait complexion, many pigmented moles, and bizarre tics or blinking eyes. Insomnia is common. Strong cravings or aversions to one or more of the following foods are common: salt, milk, eggs, meat fat, fruit. Symptoms may appear after a servere reaction to a vaccination. Often, there is a family member with cancer.

CHAMOMILE

These children have a bad temper and are very irritable and impatient. You will find them complaining, frustrated, restless, and thirsty. They do not know what they want; demands one thing then wants another. Chamomile children want to be carried everywhere or will whine and scream. Rocking calms them down. There is an aversion to be touched with a hypersensitivity to pain. An excellent name for them is "cannot bear it." They can't bear themselves, other people, pain, or other things. Everything is intolerable. There is a dullness of the senses with a diminished power of comprehension. The child understands nothing properly as if they were prevented by a sort of dullness of hearing. The symptoms also seem to worsen at night.

CINA

These are children who are often restless, fidgety and fretful, especially during sleep. They grind their teeth at night and wet the bed. Sleep is very restless, accompanied by jerking, frequent swallowing and coughing. A common sleeping position for the child is to lie on the belly or the hands and knees during sleep (Medorrhinum has this also). The nose seems irritated causing a constant desire to rub, pick, or bore into it until it bleeds. You may notice the twitching of face muscles and eyelids. This child does not want to be touched or even looked at and turns away when approached. Cina children are cross, contrary, disobedient with very difficult behavior. Nothing pleases them for long. Appetites are often ravenous, and sometimes they have large bellies. Thirst is considerable and they often want sweets. Other symptoms may include itchy ears and seizures. Parasites may be present.

HELLEBORUS

A medical history may reveal encephalitis or a head injury. Mental processes are so sluggish that these children feel stupid, feel that they cannot deal with things and act dull and unresponsive. They are unable to memorize anything or get the words out. There is a tendency to despair with a great aversion to making any effort, yet easily angered. They often bite their spoon when eating without being aware of it.

HYOSCYAMUS

These are difficult children with poor impulse control. They seem unable to think. Your questions may go unanswered or they cannot bear anyone talking to them. They are very animated seeming silly and foolish and smiling and laughing at everything. They may make ridiculous gestures like a dancing clown or monkeys. Jealousy of their siblings is common and they may injure them. Hyoscyamus children talk excessively with episodes of mania and rage that might include hitting and screaming. Depression is never far from the manic stage. This child can be a totally shameless exhibitionist and can have other bizarre behaviors that may reveal a strong sexual component, along with cursing for shock value. There is intense and violent excitability with fear, delirium, and the delusion of being poisoned. They are manipulative, lying, and violent children. Hyoscyamus children do not tolerate being covered up.

LACHESIS

These children are very jealous of siblings and tend to be vengeful, as well as sarcastic and nasty. Emotions such as severe depression, withdrawal, and hopelessness are often part of this self-destructive personality, along with a marked lack of confidence. Their self-criticism and irritability causes them to reproach themselves severely. At times, there seems no way of stopping this negative behavior. At other times they turn this behavior on others. Their aggression surfaces easily and makes them difficult to live and work with. Lachesis children are restless and their mood variable. You will find them suspicious with a marked preoccupation about others. They feel that others are often criticizing them and putting them on the defensive. Their mood may be severely agitated and hyperactive and they can talk until they become completely exhausted. They wake from sleep unrefreshed and even more agitated. This aggravation through sleep is the major diagnostic feature. They hate any kind of physical or behavioral restriction, like tight clothing or being "grounded."

LYCOPODIUM

Lycopodium children are dictatorial and bossy at home where they feel safe. In other places they may act like bullies, being cocky and boastful, but are really cowards. They are usually intelligent and good at schoolwork, but will do anything to "save face," especially to the public. These children have performance anxiety and feel insecure in all situations. You will not find them really relaxed, but fidgeting both mentally and physically. They are fearful of any new situation and intolerant of any change in mealtimes or diet. Their biggest fear is that a demand will be made of them and they are not prepared for it. Anything can be seen as a demand or a threat. They usually worry about the future. Some of their physical problems are dyslexia, digestive problems, and the desire for sweets. Other symptoms include the inability to concentrate, poor memory, and chronic fatigue.

MEDORRHINUM

These children often fear going to public places, and especially having to eat in public. Any public situation where they have to eat is dreaded. The worst disaster is always anticipated. If they cannot escape the situation, then they feel sure that they will die. They do better at the seashore. These are the types that want "drugs, sex, and rock 'n roll." Most of the time these children are aggressive and have temper tantrums, but they may be passive and emotionally withdrawn. On one hand, they love animals, but at the same time they can be malicious. They are night owls and may sleep on their abdomen with their bottom in the air. Other symptoms include restlessness, impatience, a wandering mind that cannot pay attention or finish tasks, impulsiveness, and mistakes in spelling, reading and writing. They may be hypersexual. Foods they love are unripened fruits, oranges, meat fat, and ice.

NUX VOMICA

The basic personality is irritable and aggressive with short bursts of rage and resentment that flares up and just as quickly cools down and is over. Nothing is ever done moderately or in a natural, quiet, rhythmic way. This leads to periods of tiredness and exhaustion. Sometimes confidence is lacking causing these children to suffer intently at the least slight or joking criticism. You will find them feeling inadequate, unhappy, and unsatisfied most of the time. Because of their fiery temperament, these children are impatient and frustrated. They are highly competitive and must be first and the best. They are highly critical and intolerant children and rarely ever know how to relax. Sleep is rarely satisfactory. There may be a tendency to spasm and they are overly sensitive to everything, especially noise, smells, or bright lights. The past preoccupies them rather than the present.

PLATINA OR PLATINUM

These are children (usually girls) who are arrogant and contemptuous. They have the illusion that the people around them are physically and mentally inferior. It is often a defense against feelings of failure, rejection, and a lack of confidence. They feel forsaken and unloved with a need to reconnect to people. Girls will send out a sexual message and tend to be jealous of other women. Platina children live and dwell on the past. There may be anger, indignation and paranoia. This child may have overwhelming and aggressive impulses that provoke the most severe depression and confused states. She can be so indescribably happy that she would embrace anything and laugh at the saddest thing. She can also get so sad that the most joyful things are distressing and any serious thought terrifying. This child seems out-of-sorts with the whole world. She may experience marked anxiety with trembling, as well as oppressed breathing and violent palpitation. They are very restless children and cannot remain in one spot.

STRAMONIUM

This is a remedy for terrors. Stramonium children are nervous with fears about death, the dark, dogs, evil, suffocation, and abandonment. They become overly vigilant to combat these fears and become violent if controlled. These children have a horror of glistening objects. Thirst is great, yet they dread water. Other symptoms may include nightmares and terrors that become increasingly worse between midnight and 2 a.m. Often, they wake screaming and in fear. Their symptoms seem to be even worse after they experience fright or rage. There may be breaks with reality, leading to violent and sudden mood changes. This can manifest as swings from severe hyperactivity to bouts of depression. These children are impulsive, malicious, and display bad behavior resulting in striking and biting. They spit, slam doors, and threaten to hurt people. A traumatic event or abuse may have taken place prior to the onset of symptoms. Kids may dress up as power figures.

Children needing this homeopathic remedy do not have a correct estimate of distance or size and they will reach for things that are across the room. This causes them to bump into people and things. Wrong names and wrong words are used and they cannot find the right words for things. They sit silently, eyes on the ground, picking at their clothes. Their mind wanders with quick motions of the eyes and hands. An expression of stupidity or fear presents on their face. All food taste bitter or there is a loss of taste.

SULPHUR

These children usually do not like water or being bathed. They tend to be untidy in every aspect. At night they overheat easily and stick their feet out of bed. They are opinionated and think that they are always right. Most of them are daydreamers and commonly withdraw into a fantasy world. Their perceptions and thought processes are in disorder and illogical. These children need to control and create their own boundaries in any situation, often having their own rules. Memory is poor and they experience much confusion. Any enclosed situation threatens them. Sweets and fried foods are desired.

TARANTULA HISPANICA

This remedy is for the most hyperactive of all children, usually who display extreme restlessness and impulsiveness. They love lively music and dancing, as well as bright colors. This may calm them down temporarily from their self-destructive activity. Moods change abruptly with excessive fits of laughing, singing, dancing, and screaming that may change suddenly to depression. These children have unceasing movement, constant jerking, twitching, running, and the hands and fingers are never still. Sometimes they constantly pick at their fingers or wad of bits of paper and throw them away. Their thought processes are in a state of turmoil and emotions are excessive. These children steal and lie. They are manipulative, cunning, and hypersexual, yet timid. Violence can suddenly surface with an incredible swiftness of action.

TUBERCULINUM

These restless children are deliberately destructive and malicious with anger and violence. They become indifferent to reprimands. You can find them banging their head on the wall or floor, throwing tantrums, hitting and biting others and breaking things. It is common to find them fearful, as well as allergic to cats. Milk and sugar are common cravings, but they are often allergic to milk. They love salty and smoked meats. Other symptoms include the desire for travel, a Jekyll-Hyde personality, difficulty concentrating, and grinding their teeth at night. Fatigue, faintness, and general debility have been described. They prefer the open air and want doors and windows kept open. Sleep is difficult in spite of being drowsy. These children have chronic respiratory problems and repeated infections, such as the common cold.

VERATRUM ALBUM

These are children who display senseless repetitive behavior and hyperactivity. They can be very destructive, wanting to cut up or tear to bits anything within reach. Sometimes, there is an obsessional desire to destroy things. Veratrum chidlren are restless, hurried, fidgety, and must be constantly occupied. They talk wildly and may be inconsolable over some fancied misfortune. These children tell outrageous lies, feel abandoned, and inappropriately poke, touch, hug, and kiss others. Their attitude may be condescending or superior with religious delusions. They love ice and cold drinks, lemons, and salty foods. Veratrum children often feel cold, but may sweat profusely.

Cell Salts

A key researcher investigating the many roles of minerals in the human body was Dr. W. H. Schuessler, M.D., of Oldenburg, Germany. It was fascinating to him that natural substances could cure disease. After isolating minerals from various body tissues, he knew that minerals were an integral part of the body. Twelve mineral compounds were discovered and he called them "cell salts" or "tissue salts."

As Dr. Schuessler researched the minerals further, he felt that if the body became deficient in any of these important minerals an abnormal or diseased condition occurred. He studied the various symptoms and discovered which minerals were lacking in his patients. With the proper cell salts added to the sick cells of the body, the abnormality was corrected and the body healed itself. It was also important to give the correct amount and frequency. This was the beginning of Dr. Schuessler's biochemic system of medicine.

Cell salts can be prescribed safely and are an inexpensive way for people to self-treat many of the ills that exist today. You can experiment to find out which one your child needs without fear of damaging his or her health. This 19th-century discovery is still useful for health concerns today.

How to Select Cell Salts

The success of biochemical cell salt therapy lies in accurately linking your child's symptoms with the appropriate tissue cell salt. Symptoms occur in a variety of forms and are a guide to the nature of the body's deficiency and to the correct treatment required. How and where they occur will help you decide the correct tissue cell salt. Often, there is a need for more than one. The proper dose replenishes the cell salt supply and restores tissue or organ function.

Cell salt remedies are meticulously extracted from living plants in an alcohol process. Manufacturers pulverize the natural mineral substances and blend them with milk sugar to make them more palatable. Many potencies are available, but the 3X and 6X are the best for home use. The most generally useful potency is 6X. Liquid homeopathic remedies are available from some health-care practitioners and used in a similar manner as the tablet form.

HOW TO USE CELL SALTS

The success of biochemical cell salt therapy lies in accurately linking a person's symptoms with the appropriate biochemical cell salt. Symptoms occur in a variety of forms and are a guide to the nature of the body's deficiency and to the correct treatment required. The correct balance of these cell salts must be maintained for proper structure and function of each tissue and organ. How and where the symptoms occur will help you decide the correct cell salt for your child. Often, more than one is needed.

Cell salts provide inorganic elements in a form that ensures their transportation and assimilation into the body. For the greatest effectiveness, place the tablets under the tongue and allow them to dissolve. This lets the dose of cell salts bypass the stomach, which assures that the remedy or remedies will travel quickly and undamaged to the cells that are diseased or injured. Use a clean spoon to remove them from the bottle and then place them under the tongue. For small children, it may be easier to dissolve the tablets in a little water first and then squirt the liquid inside the lip or under the tongue. If quick relief is needed, dissolve the tablets in a cup of hot water and sip often. Hold the liquid under the tongue for about a minute for maximum absorption. Never touch any of the cell salt tablets with your fingers.

Most homeopathic remedies can be stored for many years when the bottles are keep tightly closed in dry areas free from light, radiation, and away from strong odors. Substances that can cause the cell salts to become non-functional are caffeine, aromatics oils (such as mint in toothpaste) and other strong odors, and strongly spiced foods. Several other cautions are important during treatment: avoid handling the tablets because of contamination; never expose the medicines to direct sunlight; don't eat raw garlic; don't expose the cell salts to X-rays at airports; and don't sleep under electric blankets.

Biochemical cell salts can be used with perfect safety. They do not produce unwanted side effects, conflict with other medicines, and are non-addictive. Even babies and small children can take them with complete safety. The following symptoms may describe your child and the subsequent cell salt remedies may be of help. You can mix the different cell salts together. Give all the cell salt remedies listed following the indicated symptom. Continue the indicated salt(s) for several days after the symptoms clear.

Besides the dosage information given by the cell salt manufacturer, the following information can generally be followed with favorable results. Chronic cases may require you to take tablets three to four times a day. The remedy or remedies may have to be taken for a month or longer. Acute cases of sudden onset may require you to take one dose 1 to 2 hours apart and decrease frequency as symptoms improve. In acute or severe cases, take the dose every 15 minutes to an hour, and decrease frequency with improvement. With less acute cases, take the remedy hourly, and decrease the frequency as symptoms improve.

The following is a list of conditions resembling the supposed symptoms of ADD/hyperactivity and the cell salts used to treat the condition. For more information on cell salts and their specific applications, refer to my book, *Natural Healing with Cell Salts,* also published by Woodland.

Agitated....Silica
Anger, easily, with irritability....Calc Sulph, Nat Mur
Anger at trifles....Nat Phos
Anxious moods....Kali Phos
Attention difficult to fix....Silica
Brain and nerve tissue, affects....Silica, Kali Phos
Can't concentrate....Calc Phos, Silica
Changeable moods....Calc Sulph, Kali Phos
Comprehension slow....Calc Phos
Conditions with symptoms of nervousness, irritability, depression, sleeplessness....Kali Phos, Mag Phos
Crying and screaming frequently....Kali Phos, Nat Mur
Depression....Kali Phos, Nat Mur

Development, mental and physical, appears slow....Calc Phos
Discouraged....Silica, Nat Sulph, Ferr Phos
Disposition unhappy, with symptoms of fretfulness, ill-humor, laziness....Kali Phos
Dullness and unable to concentrate....Mag Phos
Exhaustion, irritable, excited....Silica
Fidgety....Kali Phos
Fits of crying....Kali Phos
Hard to think....Silica
Helps to steady the nerves....Mag Phos
Ill-tempered....Kali Phos, Calc Phos
Impatience is great....Kali Phos
Memory impaired....Calc Phos, Kali Phos
Mental faculties, helps sharpen; maintains contented disposition....Kali Phos
Nervous exhaustion....Nat Phos, Kali Phos
Obstinate....Kali Sulph
Overly sensitive....Silica, Kali Phos
Primary cell salt for children....Calc Phos
Rambling or excessive talk....Nat Mur, Kali Phos, Ferr Phos
Screaming....Kali Phos
Temper (bad)....Calc Phos, Kali Phos
Tic, usually in the face....Ferr Phos, Mag Phos
Tonic for the nerves....Nat Phos, Calc Phos, Mag Phos, Kali Phos

FLOWER ESSENCES

Flower essences are prepared by an infusion of only the flowering part of the plant in a bowl of pure spring water and then left in the open air for several hours. These flower essences represent particular "archetypal" patterns corresponding to human personality traits, emotions, attitudes and life lessons. They help to increase our awareness and to transform blocks to the full unfolding of a person's potential. It is possible to transform attitudes and emotions that hinder the full health of the individual and eventually have adverse effects on physical health.

Flower essences allow more flexibility in selection than homeopathics, with no apparent danger or harmful effect if the wrong remedy is chosen. This may account for their growing popularity across a wide range of professions, including conventional and naturopathic medicine, psychological and spiritual counseling, physical therapy, and traditional homeopathy. Flower essences should be seen in the context of an overall approach to child care that includes other supportive attention. I suggest further reading about flower essences.

Agrimony: The child appears cheerful and easy going, but is often filled with inner torment. It is hard for her to read in a group.

Aspen: These children have anxiety for no apparent reason.

California Wild Rose: The appetite is poor with a lack of interest in food and vitality is low.

Calendula: This child is a poor listener and has difficulty being receptive to what others are saying. They are often argumentative and have communication problems in relationships.

Chamomile: This is a good remedy for calming hyperactivity in children, fussiness, tension-created digestive disturbances in the stomach area, and emotional tension that interferes with learning and concentration.

Chestnut Bud: Children who have difficulty with learning experiences often need chestnut bud. These are children who often lag behind others, repeat mistakes, and have difficulty learning their lessons.

Chicory: These children have temper tantrums, demanding excessive attention usually by negative behavior. They can be overly fussy as a way of getting attention and become particularly irritable when they do not get the attention demanded. There is a tendency to cling or feel sorry for themselves.

Clematis: This is the daydreamer whose attention is elsewhere. They escape from the present by fantasizing about the future.

Cosmos: This remedy harmonizes overly active minds. These children have too many ideas flood in simultaneously so that they are unable to focus. This affects them especially when speaking.

They do not seem to have the ability to integrate thinking and speech when the mind is overwhelmed by too much information.

Dill: These children seem overwhelmed when too many experiences occur too quickly or when starting a new project. Dill is for children that seem "over-amped."

Elm: This is a good remedy over being overwhelmed and feeling over-extended and isolated.

Filaree: This flower essence helps to let go of worries and anxieties. This is for children who over-focus on details while losing the larger view.

Five-Flower Remedy or *Rescue Remedy:* Give this in extreme situations when the child is totally out of control. This combination of five remedies causes immediate centering and brings balance after extreme stress.

Gentian: This is a good remedy for children who easily give up when they encounter difficulties. It gives them the strength to persevere despite setbacks. Gentian is also good for discouragement after rejection or failure or the inability to recoup and move on.

Golden Yarrow: This flower essence is good for performance anxiety. It helps give the child confidence to perform despite the anxiety.

Goldenrod: When a child needs social approval because they are unsure of their own values, give them goldenrod. Often they create barriers to others by anti-social or obnoxious behavior.

Holly: Sibling rivalry and jealousy are often symptoms that call for holly. These children feel there is not enough love to go around. Holly helps them to let go of jealousy and envy.

Impatiens: This remedy helps overly hasty children who are also overly impulsive and restless. They become easily frustrated and quick to anger with fiery temperaments. Anger and intolerance toward others sometimes leads to violence or abuse. They have a tendency to eat too fast.

Indian Pink: When there is a desire to remain calm while being centered in the middle of intense or frenetic activity, Indian Pink is the remedy. It also seems to help focus a child when the nerves seem frazzled.

Iris: This remedy helps when there is a craving for sweets and general hypoglycemic tendencies.

Larch: Children with many emotional symptoms concerning self-confidence are helped by larch. It helps with overcoming the fear of ridicule by others, fear of failure, anxiety, self-blame, and gives confidence in self-expression or public performance.

Lavender: This remedy is for soothing frayed and over-stimulated nerves. It is for children that are too high strung and sleep too lightly.

Madia: This flower essence helps to focus attention and concentration, overcome the tendency to be distracted, increase the attention to detail, and let go of scattered thoughts.

Mallow: These are children that have difficulty making social contact with others, leading to feelings of isolation and abandonment. They have trouble maintaining friendships with others.

Mimulus: When more confidence is needed to face daily challenges and fears, then mimulus is needed.

Morning Glory: This remedy is needed when there is an addiction to junk food and stimulants such as caffeine, late-night binging, irregular habits, and nervous problems due to an erratic lifestyle.

Peppermint: This child cannot maintain mental attention. They are sleepy after eating and do not have the ability to use their mental forces adequately.

Pine: This is for the child that is always being hard on herself and filled with guilt.

Pink Monkeyflower: This child avoids social attention and wants to hide or cover-up. They create barriers out of a sense of shame, unworthiness, and feelings of vulnerability. Being highly sensitive, they do not want to be hurt. They cannot express their real feelings and hold them deep inside because they fear judgment or censure. They do not think others will accept or understand them.

Poison Oak: These children are easily irritated and impatient. They cope with hypersensitivity by showing anger or hostility. They fear contact with others and are unable to form sympathetic bonds. These children need to understand the meaning of boundaries or limits.

Quaking Grass: These have trouble listening and working with others in a group situation.

Rabbitbrush: These children do not have the ability to handle many different details or activities at one time. They seem confused by many details. Rabbitbrush helps with mental flexibility and alertness.

Rosemary: There is poor memory function. These children are sleepy and forgetful in daytime. Rosemary helps provide a greater wakefulness and vitality. It is also good for stagnant digestion.

Snapdragon: These children have a tendency to be angry and argumentative in communications with others. There is a tendency to verbal abuse with derogatory comments. They are easily set off or snap back when feeling challenged or attacked. Biting is common.

Vine: There is a tendency to put their own wishes before those of others. A child needing vine has to be in control. They are the "bully" child.

White Chestnut: This remedy helps to still the thoughts that are constantly churning; there are strong tendencies of an overactive mind.

Chapter 26

HERBAL REMEDIES

Nature has provided herbs that act as some of the best nervines, calming agents, and relaxants with little or no side effects. There are herbs which help reduce hyperactivity (and symptoms associated with ADD), all of which are widely available in natural food stores as single herbs or included in formulas. Herbs are generally bought in bulk to make teas or as finished products like capsules, tablets, or liquid extracts. The liquid extract is especially useful for children, because they can be disguised in tea or juice. Some parents add liquid herbs to applesauce or nut butter to hide the taste. These liquids work quickly (in ten to twenty minutes) compared with slower working powdered products. The appropriate children's dose can easily be regulated, depending on age and size. Never mix herbs and prescription drugs together at the same time without the advice of your physician. It can change the effect of both. Herbs can be taken without adverse effects in most cases, but the dose must be reduced for children. A rule for determining dosage is to calculate the dosage according to the body weight of the child.

- Preschool children take approximately 1/4 of the adult dosage.
- From age five through ten, 1/2 the adult dosage is sufficient.
- Early teens take 3/4 the adult dosage.
- A child reaching adult size (age 16-21) can use the full adult dose.

The following list of herbs gives information on how they are typically used to treat symptoms commonly associated with ADD/hyperactivity.

ALFALFA (MEDICAGO SATIVA)

Alfalfa leaves and seeds provide a rich nutrient source. They are high in protein and vitamin content. It also aids in eliminating toxins. Other benefits to the body affect fatigue, anemia, and nausea.

ASTRAGALUS (ASTRAGALUS HOANTCHY)

This herb is an energizer and combats fatigue by nourishing exhausted adrenal glands and by reducing toxicity in the liver. It is also a strong immune-enhancing herb and superior tonic.

BORAGE (BORAGO OFFICINALIS)

It stimulates the adrenal glands and this results in increased energy and initiative, as well as helping to ease depression. Borage is restorative to the adrenal cortex.

CATNIP (NEPETA CATARIA)

Catnip is excellent for calming the nervous system and to relieve stress and tension. It relaxes and soothes the nervous system while decreasing irritation and restlessness. It is ideal for insomnia. Catnip is wonderful for children and infants when nervousness is present and mixes well with chamomile and lemon balm.

CHAMOMILE (MATRICARIA CHAMOMILLA)

This is a nerve tonic with relaxing properties that improve mild sleep disorders. It has a profound ability to calm the nerves and reduce tension. Chamomile is one of the best herbs for treating upset stomach and indigestion. It is safe, effective, gentle and a good-tasting relaxant for children. Chamomile is a valuable drink to stimulate appetite. Give your child a cup of tea prior to bed time to calm the nervous system and promote sleep. It also contains significant amounts of calcium, magnesium, zinc, manganese, and iron.

GINGER ROOT (ZINGIBERIS OFFICINALIS)

Ginger supports the digestive and elimination systems of the body. Eating disorders and digestive disturbances often accompany nervous tension and anxiety. Ginger assists almost every aspect of digestion and will settle a nervous stomach. It also improves circulation.

GOTU KOLA (CENTELLA ASIATICA)

This herb is a central nervous system tonic that improves mental stamina, physical fatigue, and improves energy stores. It is especially helpful for proper brain function including increased concentration and memory. It improves a child's learning ability by facilitating better recall. Anxiety can be reduced because of this herb's calming effect. It helps relieve depression and maintains stable blood sugar levels.

HOPS (HUMULUS LUPULUS)

Hops have a sedative and calming effect on the nervous system that helps with restlessness, particularly associated with anxiety. It is used to treat hyperactivity, irritability and nervous exhaustion. It helps with insomnia and nightmares. Another use of hops has been to fill a muslin pillow with it to help provide non-drug-induced sleep. Hops are known for relaxing excited cerebral conditions. Take hops in the evening. It is also good for a nervous stomach and poor appetite.

KAVA KAVA (PIPER METHYSTICUM)

People note a sense of well-being when consuming kava kava as a drink. Use it in the treatment of nervous anxiety and restlessness and for those needing an improvement in their mood. This herb calms nervousness and helps to fight fatigue. As an herbal muscle relaxant and nervous system relaxant, it invokes sleep.

KELP (LAMINARIA, FUCUS, OR SARGASSUM SPP.)

Kelp provides organic iodine that promotes healthy thyroid function that might be associated with depression, lethargy, and general malaise. The iodine content of this plant is important for thyroid disorders, whether underactive or overactive. It feeds the thyroid that in turn controls metabolism. Kelp is a glandular balancer. It also contains vitamins and minerals and cell salts considered vital to health. It helps to balance the effects of stress, provide nutritional support to the nervous system, and normalize brain function. Kelp's other trace elements can assist in various metabolic processes in the body, as well as carbohydrate metabolism.

LAVENDER (LAVANDULA SPP.)

Lavender is a natural relaxant useful for treating nervous exhaustion and alleviating mental strain. Put lavender into a warm bath one hour before bedtime. This can help relax the body and promote sleep.

LEMON BALM (MELISSA OFFICINALIS)

This is a great lemon-tasting herb, especially for children and infants. Combine it with catnip tea for nervous and hyperactive children with digestive disturbances. Lemon balm is widely used to treat depression and symptoms that are the result of stress. It has a mild relaxing effect.

PASSIONFLOWER (PASSIFLORA INCARNATA)

Passionflower is used extensively as a cerebral relaxant and relieves cerebral irritation. It is a natural tranquilizer to relax the body and mind. Passionflower works well in formulas designed to treat insomnia, but it works even better in formulas designed to combat stress, nervous tension, anxiety, restlessness, irritability, hyperactivity, and nervous headaches. It is quieting and soothing to the nervous system. It is also a good for exhaustion and muscle twitching. Problems with concentration in school children and decreased motor-nerve activity are helped with this herb. It may not be suitable for young children.

RED CLOVER BLOSSOM (TRIFOLIUM PRATENSE)

This herb is high in vitamin A. It also has value in the relief of nervous tension and as a cleanser of body toxins. It is an excellent choice in any tea blend because it is a blood purifier, as well as a gentle nerve relaxant. Red clover tea can be used over a long period of time. It is used as a nerve tonic for delicate children.

ROSEMARY (ROSMARINUS OFFICINALIS)

This herb assists in combating stress and improves the memory. Rosemary is of great benefit as a substitute for aspirin in treating headaches. It is high in assimilable calcium and a benefit to the entire nervous system.

SCHIZANDRA (SCHISANDRA CHINENSIS)

Schizandra is known as a relaxant to the body and helpful in treating forgetfulness. It works with Siberian ginseng to combat stress and support sugar levels and liver function. It also increases the energy supply of cells in the brain, muscles, and nerves. Schizandra helps to build the body's immune system and support the body against damage due to stress. It is a stress tonic for nervous disorders. Use it to treat insomnia and exhaustion, as well as to increase mental alertness and energy.

SKULLCAP (SCUTELLARIA LATERIFLORA)

Skullcap has proven itself useful for insomnia, restless sleep, nightmares, tremors and spasms. This herb is used in nearly all herbal combinations that treat nervous disorders, such as nervous irritations, exhaustion, weakness, and agitation. As a relaxant, it helps calm the mind and nervous system. It has a soothing and relaxing effect that quiets the person and brings about natural sleep. Skullcap is a slow but sure remedy for most nervous disorders. It must be taken regularly over a long period of time to be of permanent benefit. It is an excellent nerve tonic giving the feeling of well-being and inner calm. Use this herb as fresh as possible since much of its activity is lost with prolonged storage. When skullcap is combined with wood betony, lavender, and lemon balm, its calming effect is enhanced. It is not recommended for children under six years of age.

SIBERIAN GINSENG (ELEUTHEROCOCCUS SPP.)

This herb supports the immune system as well as improves energy levels, stamina, mental function, and reduces mental fatigue. It is a good stress fighter, helping the body maintain proper function when subjected to a stressful environment. It is very important to nervous system function whether it be hypoactive or hyperactive. People using ginseng are better at withstanding adverse conditions. Mental stressors such as depression and anxiety are helped by increasing a sense of well-being. Ginseng supports adrenal function and regulates blood sugar. It has a protective effect on the adrenal and thyroid glands. Stress can over excite the nervous system and induce glandular dysfunction. It will raise blood pressure. It protects the body against the effects of toxic chemicals and radiation.

The Korean and Chinese variety of ginseng are preferred in North America. Chinese ginseng has a tonic effect on the pituitary gland and a stimulating effect on the adrenal glands. Siberian ginseng helps in many nervous disorders and helps with mental or physical exhaustion. It curbs irritability and improves appetite, sleep, and chronic anxiety.

ST. JOHN'S WORT (HYPERICUM PERFORATUM)

This is the best herb for treating mild to moderate depression, including depressive states, fear, and other nervous disturbances. Use it as a sedative, and also with bedwetting and muscular twitching. St. John's wort is a natural mood elevator promoting improvement of mental outlook, alleviating anxiety and feelings of worthlessness, and improving sleep quality.

VALERIAN (VALERIANA OFFICINALIS)

This is one of the best nerve tonics and relaxants of the central nervous system. Valerian is probably the most widely used botanical for nervous tension and anxiety. It also improves alertness and the ability to concentrate. Use it for depression, as a natural sedative to improve sleep quality and relieve insomnia. It stabilizes the nervous system and increases physical and mental performance while relieving symptoms of restlessness and stress.

Unfortunately, valerian root has an unpleasant odor. The scent is hard to ignore. Use valerian according to recommended dosages. It is excellent as a tea, fresh plant liquid, or powdered extract. It is not recommended for prolonged use, but is considered safe in prescribed doses.

WILD LETTUCE (LACTUCA SPP.)

This is a safe and mild sleep aid and sedative. You usually see it mixed with other herbs in a formula. It is often used to treat nervous disorders and calm restlessness and anxiety.

WILD OAT (AVENA SATIVA)

Wild oat is a gently stimulating nervine tonic and cerebral restorative. It is indicated for nervous irritation, such as in hyperactivity. Wild oat is high in vitamin C and the B-complex vitamins. It also works as an antidepressant and restorative nerve tonic. Do not use if you have a gluten intolerance.

WOOD BETONY (STACHYS OFFICINALIS)

Wood betony has been well appreciated and prescribed for hundreds of years for treating nervous and sleep disorders. Wood betony helps to promote feelings of emotional stability and is also good for anxiety or irritability. It also helps with indigestion and stomach cramps.

HERBAL TEAS

Instead of soft drinks (many are loaded with sugar) or bottled fruit juices that contain a considerable amount of fructose, there are a number of delicious herbal teas. Instead of using sugar, sweeten the teas with stevia and licorice, or with apple juice. Try herbal teas such as chamomile, peppermint, spearmint, orange peel, cinnamon, and hibiscus. Try adding a small handful of fresh spearmint or peppermint leaves to the final blend. Drink the tea hot, chilled, or make it into popsicles by pouring into molds and freezing. A tea found to be very effective for calming hyperactive children is a combination of passionflower, valerian, skullcap, hops, licorice, and catnip.

Chapter 27

⌐

NUTRITIONAL
SUPPLEMENTS

D octors seldom stay up to date on all the new healing compounds and methods of treatment. There are only so many
hours in a day and a busy conventional doctor is often
hard-pressed just to keep up on the new drugs. Even if they were
interested in alternative and natural treatments, they usually do not
have the time to study about breakthroughs in herbs, homeopathic
remedies, supplements, or nutritional treatments. We have millions
of children who have mental and emotional problems. A large number of them could benefit from nutritional treatment.

Parents should use caution when self-treating without the guidance from a health professional trained in nutrition. There are many
products available today and confusing information abounds. With
the proper guidance, you and your child can succeed. Supplements
that may be helpful for ADD, hyperactivity, and other learning disabilities may include those found in the following list. These supplements generally help with symptoms and conditions associated with
ADD and hyperactivity.

Mineral Deficiencies

Minerals are arguably the most important of all the body's nutrients. Vitamins, proteins, enzymes, and amino acids, as well as fats and carbohydrates, require minerals for activity. Trace minerals such as zinc, copper, and chromium are only needed in small or trace amounts by the body, but they are no less important to the functioning of the body than the other "macro" minerals: calcium, magnesium, potassium, sulphur, etc. There are eighty-four known minerals, with seventeen being essential. If there is a shortage of just one of them, the balance of the body's systems can be thrown off. More and more people are suffering from mineral deficiencies as minerals continue to disappear from our soils and food supply.

Tables showing the nutrient content of foods can no longer be relied upon because minerals are disappearing faster than updated charts can be published. There is even a great variation in mineral content of foods grown in different locations and under different conditions. Modern "agribusiness" farming methods, including the widespread use of nitrogen-phosphorous-potassium fertilizer, over-farming, and loss of humus, are some factors that deplete foods.

When trace minerals are scarce in plant bodies, they are also scarce in human bodies. These deficient plants also tend to be deficient in vitamins and in protein. It is primarily the amino acid component of protein that forms neurotransmitters. These neurotransmitters have a huge amount to do with mental functioning. Correction of mineral and nutritional imbalances often causes dramatic improvement in sleep patterns, concentration, and the ability to interact socially in a normal manner. Refer to the following list for information on the main minerals and their nutrtional uses.

Calcium

This mineral is certainly important for good health, especially if one gets little sunshine or eats a poor diet, low-fat diet, or has malabsorption. Diets high in sodium, sugar, caffeine, and protein, along with low exercise, are primary causes of calcium imbalances.

Calcium is for bone and teeth metabolism, heart rhythm regularity, nerve transmission, muscle growth, muscle contraction, and cell membrane balance. Calcium should be balanced with magnesium for proper nerve function and for a healthy body. Calcium, magnesium, and zinc have a calming effect on the body. Take before bedtime to help relax muscles and promote sleep.

If your child craves milk and dairy products, this may indicate that your child is low in calcium and is having trouble absorbing the calcium from the dairy products. Add calcium supplements and avoid dairy products. Calcium needs adequate stomach acid to be metabolize adequately. Do not give your child antacids that contain calcium. Symptoms of a deficiency may include muscle cramps, arm and leg numbness, sensitivity to noise, tooth decay, as well as tingling of the lips, tongue, fingers, and feet.

CHROMIUM

This mineral is required for regulating blood sugar levels. Many hyperactive children are sugar and carbohydrate intolerant which leads to severe mood swings. Chromium is needed to make insulin more efficient in carbohydrate metabolism. Symptoms of a deficiency include glucose intolerance, weight loss, and mental confusion.

COPPER

Copper can be present in toxic amounts in body tissues, and at the same time be unavailable for physiological use. This condition is known as bio-unavailability and can occur when there is adrenal insufficiency. In some hyperactive and learning disabled children with elevated hair copper levels, the copper is not available and must be given as a supplement in order to obtain optimum results. Understanding the concept of bio-unavailability can resolve the paradox of a person having toxic copper levels and yet need to take copper supplements. This mineral is needed for iron metabolism, hemoglobin synthesis, and neurotransmitter formation. Symptoms of a deficiency include anemia, low white blood cell count, bone spurs, depigmentation, weak nails, low body temperature, and sparse, brittle or kinky hair.

IODINE

Iodine is necessary for the proper function of the thyroid gland which controls metabolism. The thyroid gland then helps to facilitate energy production and physical and mental development. A deficiency can cause cold hands and feet, dry hair and skin, irritability, nervousness, obesity, constipation, dermatitis, swollen fingers and toes, and hypothyroidism. A low thyroid can cause additional symptoms of fatigue, lethargy, and a mind that is slow and dull.

IRON

An iron deficiency in children can produce symptoms that look like ADD, such as decreased attentiveness and persistent activity. Guatemalan infants with iron deficiency have been shown to score lower on the Bayley Scale of Mental Development. Preschool iron-deficient children are less likely to pay attention to relevant cues in problem-solving situations. Introducing iron back into the diet or as a supplement is likely to result in improvement. Iron is needed if the diet is high in phosphorus or there is low stomach acid. Other reasons to take iron are poor diet and times of rapid growth. Symptoms of a deficiency include constipation, skin pallor, fatigue, confusion, depression, dizziness, cold hands and feet, headaches, anorexia, irritability, brittle concave nails, sore tongue, pain in the hands and feet, heart palpitations, low stomach acid, skin sores, fragile bones, eating ice or dirt, gas, nausea, and stomach distress with belching.

LITHIUM

In a study of thirty-eight aggressive, hyperactive, combative, unstable and mentally retarded children, sixty-three percent had a sharp reduction in the frequency of their aggressive behavior after receiving lithium in their drinking water. Possible signs of a deficiency may be manic-depressive disorder and other nervous and mental disorders.

MAGNESIUM

If your child craves chocolate there is a good chance they need more magnesium. Take away the chocolate and give the child magnesium along with daily calcium. Calcium and magnesium have a calming effect and are best taken before bedtime. Calcium levels tend to be low if your child is on a poor diet with no green vegetables, nuts, or seeds. Deficiencies are common in times of stress or when there is diarrhea, diabetes, kidney disease, or malabsorption. Symptoms of a deficiency include apathy, irritable nerves and muscles, apprehension, weakness, confusion, depression, hyperactivity, paranoia, anorexia, nausea, vomiting, sensitivity to noise, irregular heart beat, being ticklish, muscle cramps and twitches in the feet and legs, insomnia, hypothermia, hand tremors, and body odor.

MANGANESE

This mineral is needed for carbohydrate metabolism, growth, energy production, and for increasing the diameter of bone growth. It is also vital for proper brain function, muscles and nerves. Some of the mental symptoms include being disagreeable, crying spells, wanting to be left alone, and seizures. Symptoms of a deficiency also include weight loss, facial tics, dermatitis, nausea, vomiting, changes in hair color, dizziness, muscle coordination problems, low cholesterol, injures easily, strained knees, loss of hearing, poor bone growth, bone deformities, and the slow growth of hair and nails.

MOLYBDENUM

There is a need for this mineral in enzyme system functions. It is particularly involved in the oxidation process that is considered antagonistic to copper being protective in copper poisoning. Molybdenum is also necessary for proper carbohydrate metabolism.

PHOSPHORUS

Phosphorus is closely associated with calcium and vitamin D in the body. Most of it is in the skeleton. The rest is involved in practically every complex activity of protein, fats, and carbohydrate metabolism. Phosphorus helps to produce energy, builds new tissues, and maintain good structure. Some of the symptoms produced when there is not enough phosphorus include being fearful of the future and the unknown, bone pain, insomnia, decayed teeth, fatigue, loss of appetite, weight loss, irregular breathing, and nervous disorders.

If the phosphorus intake is too great for a child's calcium intake, then the phosphorus has nothing to combine with for absorption and is then excreted through the urine from the blood or the skeleton. Phosphorus levels can become too high by drinking too much soda pop, not consuming meat products, lack of vitamin D, milk allergy, and stress. Additionally, the use of the following substances can decrease phosphorus levels to detrimental numbers: aspirin, thyroid medication, cortisone drugs, and antacids.

POTASSIUM

Potassium is needed if your child is on a low-fruit and vegetable diet, on diuretics, or on a high-sodium diet. Penicillin treatment can cause a deficiency of potassium. Symptoms of a deficiency include muscular weakness and soreness, twitches, colic in infants, erratic and rapid heart beats, fatigue, insomnia, eczema, glucose intolerance, nervousness, and high cholesterol. Normal heart and muscle function, transmission of nerve impulses, and growth need adequate potassium balance.

SELENIUM

This mineral is an antioxidant and needed for DNA metabolism, immune function, cell membrane integrity, and pancreatic function. It helps to protect the body from the toxicity of drugs and heavy metals such as mercury and cadmium.

SODIUM

Sodium is very essential, but most people get too much, not too little. It helps maintain fluid levels in each cell and controls fluid pressure between the cells and the biological environment that surrounds them. It also helps direct the flow of other nutrients to and from the cells. If there is excess perspiration, inability of sodium utilization, as well as adrenal gland exhaustion, there may be a deficiency. Symptoms of a deficiency could include: adrenal gland exhaustion, bloating, bad breath, confusion of the mind, constipation, excessive thirst, exhaustion, hay fever, hysterical behavior, indigestion, temper tantrums, loss of smell, mental depression, fatigue, low blood pressure, and flatulence.

ZINC

If your child is diagnosed with copper toxicity then additional zinc will usually help. Supplementing with zinc is especially helpful if your child is on a low-zinc diet or commonly eats unleavened bread. A deficiency of zinc may be associated with learning disabilities and behavioral disturbances. These children are irritable, tearful, and sullen. They are not soothed by close body contact and resent disturbances. Photophobia is present and gaze aversion is common. Symptoms of a deficiency also include anemia, depression, low immunity, iron deficiency, poor growth, delayed sexual maturation, anorexia, acne, distorted taste sensation, diarrhea, apathy, birth defects, slow growing and brittle nails and hair, hair loss, eczema, fatigue, high cholesterol, poor wound healing, malabsorption, memory loss, white spots on the nails.

A zinc deficiency may allow aluminum to get into the brain. Zinc is a vital component of enzymes in the brain that repair worn-out cells. The brain needs zinc to make many enzymatic reactions occur. This mineral is also needed in healing (repair), and for proper taste, hearing, and vision. Cadmium may be elevated in behavior disturbed children. Cadmium displaces zinc in biochemical reactions or halts processes normally catalyzed by zinc. Adequate zinc may protect against the adverse effects of cadmium.

VITAMIN DEFICIENCIES

Dr. Nathan Masor's *The New Psychiatry* cites many examples of the effectiveness of treating mental symptoms with high doses of vitamins. Dr. Linus Pauling blamed the deficiencies of vitamin B-1, nicotinic acid, B-6, B-12, biotin, vitamin C, and folic acid for disorders of the brain and the nervous system, and mental illness. Cognitive disturbances in children may result from inadequate supplies of some minerals. A vitamin B-12 deficiency may cause severe psychiatric symptoms that may vary in severity from a mild disorder or moods to paranoid behavior. A significant number of hyperactive individuals are suffering from vitamin deficiencies or they may require more than an individual would otherwise need. It is important to discuss any vitamin therapy with a physician who has training in nutrition. The following vitamins may be helpful for learning disabilities and hyperactivity.

VITAMIN A

Too much vitamin A can be toxic, whereas beta-carotene is non-toxic and is converted to vitamin A in the body on an "as-needed" basis. Vitamin A assists in retinal (eye) function, tissue repair, RNA synthesis, and cell membrane balance. In addition to being a source of vitamin A, beta-carotene has a major antioxidant function in the tissues of the body. As an antioxidant, it helps build proper immune function and prevent allergies. A deficiency of vitamin A could include these symptoms: loss of appetite, blemishes, dry hair, fatigue, itching and burning eyes, loss of smell, night blindness, rough dry skin, sinus trouble, soft tooth enamel, susceptibility to infections.

B-COMPLEX

This complex of vitamins works together to calm the nervous system and support correct brain function, as well as improve concentration and memory. Specific B-vitamins including thiamine (B-1), riboflavin (B-2), niacin (B-3), pyridoxine (B6), pantothenic acid, and choline, are required for optimal nervous system function, optimal energy production, and proper sugar metabolism. When these nutrients are deficient due to inadequate dietary intake or increased demand, it can significantly contribute to hyperactive behavior. One hundred children with ADD were given megadoses of various B-complex vitamins and 15 percent responded better to pyridoxine (B-6), 8 percent to thiamine (B-1) and several to niacinamide (B-3). Half of those who benefited from pyridoxine were worse on thiamine and visa versa.

Children under stress need more B-vitamins since they are essential for maintaining good mental health. B-vitamins are vital in the production of serotonin, a chemical in the body that influences behavior. Symptoms of low B-complex vitamins could include: acne, anemia, constipation, high cholesterol, digestive disturbances, fatigue, dull and dry hair, insomnia, and rough and dry skin.

Some studies show that individual B-vitamins may antagonize the therapeutic effects of others, such as in the case of thiamine (B-1) and pyridoxine (B-6). This seems to be especially true when treating ADD. Megadoses of vitamin B-6 are capable of inducing folic acid deficiency. Keep this in mind when using vitamin B-6.

VITAMIN B-1 (THIAMINE)

Adding vitamin B-1 and eliminating a junk food diet have benefited children who show evidence of thiamine deficiency. Their behavior includes being impulsive, irritable, sensitive to criticism, easily angered, and excessively aggressive. This vitamin is needed for blood cell metabolism, digestion (acid production), energy, growth, muscle metabolism, pain inhibition, and autonomic nervous system function.

VITAMIN B-2 (RIBOFLAVIN)

Vitamin B-2 is needed if processed food are prominent in the diet, as well as stress, trauma, a need for high energy, or antibiotic use. This vitamin is also needed for antibody formation, cell respiration, red blood cell formation, and fat and carbohydrate metabolism. If a person is low in riboflavin they might have some of the following symptoms: fatigue, weight loss, depression, dizziness, photophobia, red cracked lips, burning eyelids, dermatitis, or magenta-colored tongue.

VITAMIN B-3 (NIACIN/NIACINAMIDE)

This vitamin can help normalize behavior, especially if your child eats lots of sugar and starches, does strenuous exercise, has a trauma or a rapid growth spurt, or uses antibiotics. Vitamin B-3 is needed for fat metabolism, circulation, acid production, sex-hormone metabolism, and histamine activation. Symptoms of low B-3 include: fatigue, confusion, depression, irritability, loss of sense of humor, paranoia, hypoglycemia, memory loss, crying jags, anorexia, stomach problems, diarrhea, tender gums, red and scaly dermatitis, high cholesterol, headaches, ringing in the ears, insomnia, unmanageable hair, canker sores, sore and red tongue, low stomach acid, and bad breath. There is evidence that B-3 in the form of nicotinamide helps with hyperactivity, deteriorating school performance, perceptual changes and the inability to acquire or maintain social relationships. Give it along with ascorbic acid.

VITAMIN B-6 (PYRIDOXINE)

B-6 is needed if the child has a poor diet, has infections, gets radiation, or is experiencing excessive stress. The body needs this vitamin for antibody formation, DNA/RNA synthesis, fat and protein metabolism, hemoglobin function, nerve cell metabolism, and tryptophan metabolism. Symptoms of a deficiency might include: poor memory and dream recall, fatigue, muscle weakness, irritability, nervousness, depression, dizziness, numbness, pain, tingling, headaches, low blood sugar, dandruff, seborrhea, eczema, premenstrual syndrome, asthma, allergies, anemia, stiff joints, conjunctivitis, poor wound healing, and hyperactivity.

A case report of a child with ADD receiving 3 grams of nicotinamide (B-3) daily and 0.5 grams of pyridoxine (B-6) daily had marked improvement. Vitamin B-6 helps to remove excess copper from the body if it is not needed. However, a study suggests that megadoses of vitamin B-6 may be capable of inducing a folic acid deficiency. Keep this in mind when giving large doses of vitamin B-6.

Vitamin B-6 helps with depression by raising the level of certain brain chemicals in hyperactive children, and produces a calming effect. Large amounts are vital in the production of serotonin, a chemical in the body that influences behavior. Children with ADD, who also have normal blood serotonin levels, may not benefit from megavitamin therapy, but children with low whole blood serotonin levels have been helped by B-6. In cases when B-6 was administered to hyperactive children with low serotonin levels, serotonin increased to normal and the hyperactivity disappeared.

VITAMIN B-12 (COBALAMIN)

A strict vegetarian, a chronic laxative user, or someone who has heavy bleeding will need to supplement with vitamin B-12. Vitamin B-12 is needed for blood cell formulation, appetite stimulation, cell longevity, iron absorption, and fat-protein-carbohydrate metabolism.

Symptoms of a deficiency include: weakness, fatigue, depression, irritability, memory loss, confusion, headaches, dizziness, moodiness, malabsorption, numbness and tingling, beefy red tongue, anorexia, constipation, body odor, palpitations, yellow pallor to skin, and paranoia.

BIOTIN

Biotin facilitates cell growth, fatty acid production, and protein-fat-carbohydrate metabolism. Biotin is needed if your child has a poor diet, is under excessive stress, or if malabsorption is present. Symptoms of low biotin levels include: fatigue, depression, scaly and gray-looking dermatitis or other skin conditions, a smooth magenta-colored tongue, insomnia, muscle pains, nausea, vomiting, infections, anemia, and high cholesterol.

CHOLINE

Choline stimulates acetylcholine, a calming neurotransmitter. This B-vitamin is needed if your child has a poor diet, malabsorption, or is under excessive stress. It is essential for metabolism, nerve transmission, and cell membrane function. Symptoms of low choline levels include: poor memory, confusion, vagueness, high cholesterol, heart arrhythmias, fat intolerance, gastric ulcers, growth retardation, liver impairment, kidney disease, and eczema.

PARA AMINOBENZOIC ACID (PABA)

This B-vitamin is needed if your child eats poorly or has malabsorption. It facilitates blood cell formation, protein metabolism, and growth promoting factors. Symptoms might include vitiligo, anemia, eczema, constipation, digestive disorders, fatigue, arthritis, depression, irritability, and nervousness.

PANTOTHENIC ACID

Children with poor diets, malabsorption, excessive stress, and who are on cortisone-like drugs, need pantothenic acid to help normalize behavior. It is needed for the normal functioning of tissues and muscles and protects all membranes from infections. Pantothenic acid is essential for detoxification, energy conversion, natural cortisone production, and growth stimulation. It is an antihistamine and needed for vitamin D utilization. Symptoms of a deficiency could include: impaired coordination, faintness on arising, joint and muscle pain, fatigue, depression, digestive problems, loss of appetite, constipation, insomnia, physical weakness, asthma, allergies, and irritability.

VITAMIN C

This antistress, antioxidant vitamin may help because hyperactivity is often linked to allergies and allergic conditions. Allergies frequently respond to high doses of vitamin C. This vitamin is essential for healing and in the synthesis of neurotransmitters in the brain. Vitamin C with bioflavonoids helps with adrenal and immune function. More of this vitamin is needed if your child is exposed to cigarette smoke or other pollutants. The following conditions usually call for an increase of vitamin C: injuries, fevers, infections, excessive physical activity, burns, antibiotic use, drugs, addictions, cortisone use, or anemia. Vitamin C is essential for oxygen metabolism, preventing vascular damage, helping iron absorption, and red blood cell formation, as well as helping with resistance to shock and infections.

VITAMIN D

Vitamin D (from fish oil) is needed if there is a lack of sunshine, a low-fat diet, or a high-phosphorus diet (meat and soft drinks). Vitamin D may be low during adolescence, when on a vegan diet, or if someone has malabsorption. It is necessary for calcium and phosphorous metabolism, heart action, blood clotting, and skin respiration. Symptoms of a deficiency could include soft nails, irritability, nervousness, insomnia, muscle cramps, joint pain, increased cavities, burning mouth and throat, diarrhea, and a sweaty scalp.

VITAMIN E (TOCOPHEROL)

This vitamin has been helpful for hyperactive children with learning disabilities to calm them down and make them teachable. It has been effective in eliminating bedwetting. Vitamin E may normalize brain function and protect glands during stress. It is needed if your child is exposed to pollutants, drugs, excessive stress, and vigorous exercise. Vitamin E dosages may need to be increased if there is chronic indigestion, a processed food diet, and chronic laxative use. Vitamin E is an antioxidant and is needed for blood clotting, cholesterol metabolism, capillary wall strength, lung metabolism, muscle and nerve maintenance, and detoxification. Symptoms of a deficiency could include: anemia, diabetes, elevated cholesterol, ulcerative colitis, ulcers, malabsorption, muscle swelling or wasting, brittle hair or hair that falls out excessively, and diseases of the liver, kidneys, and pancreas.

FOLIC ACID

Folic acid is necessary for the stability of the nervous system, but is destroyed by drugs like phenobarbital. These drugs are often given to young children who are hyperactive or who have seizures. Folic acid is needed if your child is not eating leafy vegetables or has parasites. It is also needed for conditions that involve bleeding, cancer, excessive stress, malabsorption, or diarrhea. Any condition resulting in the increase need for blood formation will need folic acid. Folic acid is necessary for DNA/RNA production, stomach acid production, cell reproduction and growth, appetite stimulation, nucleic acid formulation, and stability of the nervous system. Symptoms of a deficiency include: smooth and sore red tongue, mouth ulcers, dizziness, apathy, forgetfulness, anorexia, growth retardation, numbness, weakness, and restless legs.

GABA (GAMMA-AMINO BUTYRIC ACID)

This substance has been shown to help decrease hyperactivity in children as well as benefiting children with learning disabilities.

MISCELLANEOUS SUPPLEMENTS

AMINO ACIDS

A number of dietary deficiencies can result in lowered levels of the brain amines needed to maintain a healthy, optimistic mental attitude. Amino acids and vitamins have a direct impact on how children behave and whether they feel like whistling or withdrawing. The way many prescription drugs treat depression is by raising the quantity of certain brain amino acids.

DIGESTIVE ENZYMES

Some food-sensitive children produce insufficient gastric acid. This can lead to the poor absorption of nutrients such as calcium and iron. If this is the problem, eat protein foods at different times from carbohydrates. The body cannot absorb B-12 and folic acid, the essential amino acids, and minerals without sufficient hydrochloric acid. Symptoms could include digestive problems, foul-smelling gas, belching, inability to digest protein, slow bowel motility, food sensitivities, parasites, anemia, soft nails, and thin hair. Many children, especially asthmatics, are low in hydrochloric acid, especially before the age of seven. Other digestive enzymes may be involved.

DMAE (DIMETHYLAMINOETHANOL)

This substance is present in small amounts in the brain. It occurs naturally in seafood such as sardines and anchovies. Some of the brain-enhancement effects are elevated mood, improvement of memory and learning, increasing intelligence, and increased physical energy. Many people use it for its mild, safe stimulant effect. They also report that they feel less fatigue during the day and sleep better at night. DMAE is different from the stimulant effect of substances such as coffee, amphetamines, and other stimulant drugs. There is no drugged feeling or side effects common with some other drugs, nor is there depression or let-down occurs when discontinued.

There are some precautions that need to be noted. Overuse or doses that are too high can produce insomnia, dull headaches and muscle tenseness, especially of the jaws, legs, and neck. These effects completely disappear if the dosage is lowered slightly. There have not been any reports of adverse effects with DMAE. Physicians should monitor closely anyone who has epilepsy. Do not use DMAE if a person has been diagnosed with manic depression because it seems to increase the symptoms of depression. Initially, DMAE is started at low dosages with a gradual build-up to 500 to 1000 milligrams a day. Sometimes, lower dosages can result in a good response. It may take as long as three weeks to take effect.

This product is considered a nutritional supplement and available at health food stores or drug stores. It comes in bulk powder, capsules, or liquid. The liquid form of DMAE spoils without refrigeration or if left open. It needs to be kept tightly sealed in the refrigerator. Other names include: Acumen, Atrol, Bimanol, Cervoxan, Deaner, Diforene, Dimethaen, Elevan, Pabenol, Dimethylaminoethanol, Paxanol, Risatarun, Tonibral, and Varesal.

Riker Labs developed a prescription drug called Deaner or Deanol, but it is no longer available in the U.S. It had similar effects as DMAE. Riker Labs marketed their DMAE-like product for learning problems, shortened attention span, hyperactivity, under-achievement, reading and speech difficulties, impaired motor coordination, and behavior problems in children. This "smart" drug works by accelerating the brain's synthesis of the neurotransmitter acetylcholine that plays a key role in maximizing mental ability.

ESSENTIAL FATTY ACIDS (EFAS)

Studies of hyperactive children reveal that almost two-thirds of the participants show improvement after taking evening primrose oil (EPO), one of the essential fatty acids. Some children respond better to EPO if it is rubbed into their skin. This may be because of poor intestinal tract absorption. Children, usually boys, who have the most symptoms of ADD, are also the most deficient in EFAs.

The British Hyperactive Children's Support Group endorses supplementing with EFAs because they believe that hyperactive children suffer from a deficiency. They use primrose oil, either orally or rubbed into the skin, and have had remarkable results. Children that have been disruptive in school change their behavior dramatically after the use of this oil. And some children, after treatment with EFAs, can again eat foods that they were once unable to, such as wheat, with no ill effects (*Medical Hypotheses,* May 1981). Other studies of hyperactive children reveal that almost two-thirds of the participants show improvement after six to eight weeks. There have been promising improvements in behavior and function by using evening primrose oil. This therapy did not help all the children, especially those without a history of asthma, allergies, or eczema.

MENTAT

Mentat, a product from Metagenics, Inc., has had positive results in treating the symptoms of ADD. The whole herbal formulation works together to stimulate memory, reduce mental irritability, anxiety, depression, aggressiveness, and stubbornness. It helps a person to adapt to environmental and emotional stresses, stresses of school examinations and over-work. It improves the ability to concentrate and helps to rehabilitate those with behavioral disorders and disabilities in language and learning, and to some extent mental retardation of a mild to moderate degree.

Adding a multiple vitamin and mineral supplement, or a natural supplement (like those discussed in the "Miscellaneous Supplements" section) to the healing program can be one of the most simple and effective ways of relieving many of the conditions or symptoms supposedly caused by ADD. Special care must be made to ensure that the child is not sensitive to any of the supplemental products discussed in this chapter. Stay away from artificially colored and sweetened multiple vitamin and mineral supplements, and do not buy supplements that do not disclose all the ingredients on the bottle.

PYCNOGENOL

This is the trade name for proanthocyanidin, a special family of bioflavonoids. Pycnogenol is a non-toxic, water soluble nutrient. Pycnogenol holds promise as an alternative to Ritalin. Its primary mechanism of action appears to be that of a powerful antioxidant that scavenges harmful free-radicals generated by foreign toxic chemicals and possibly by other sources. Pycnogenol comes from grape seed extract or from the bark of the French maritime pine tree. Most of the research has been on the grape seed extract. Pycnogenol is not a drug and is now readily available without a prescription. Many children with ADD have found this substance effective to decrease their symptoms by normalizing brain function. It seems to improve memory by improving circulation to the brain. Free radicals reprogram DNA and are implicated in more than sixty diseases.

It has been thought to help in inflammation of the joints and other tissues, as well as improve functioning of the circulatory, nervous and immune systems.

Chapter 28

Ḡ

ADDITIONAL TREATMENTS

NUTRITIONAL THERAPIES

DETOXIFICATION

The current approach to detoxification is to nourish the body thoroughly, fueling its natural detoxification mechanism with the nutrients needed to achieve optimal detoxification activity. By providing high-quality protein, complex carbohydrates and essential fats, the body gets what it needs to prevent muscle and organ breakdown and depleted energy resources. A child needs nutrients to support the function of the organs directly involved in detoxification: intestinal tract, liver, kidneys, and fatty tissue. Intelligent application of nutrition may help in the following ways:

• *Intestine:* zinc, pantothenic acid, the amino acid L-glutamine, carbohydrates known as fructooligosaccharides (FOS), and the microorganisms *L. acidophilus* and *L. bifidus,* are a few of the substances that provide support for the health and integrity of the intestinal system. In a proper state of health, the intestine promotes elimination of toxins through regular bowel movements and providing a strong and intact barrier to prevent the leaking of toxic materials from the intestines into the circulation.

- *Liver:* The vitamins A, B-3, B-6, C, E, beta carotene, the amino acids L-cysteine, L-glutamine, and glutathione, and phospholipids, are some of the substances that support liver function. In a proper state of function, the liver filters out and transforms toxic substances that have entered the blood into harmless substances that can be excreted in the urine. Interestingly, it appears that the ratio of dietary protein to carbohydrates may be a very important factor in determining the ability of the liver to detoxify certain substances.

- *Kidney:* Vitamins A, C, B-6, and the minerals magnesium and potassium are just some of the substances that support kidney activity. The kidney provides a major route of toxin excretion in the urine.

- *Fat:* Weight reduction and management are helpful for those who are overweight. Excess fat provides a ready storage site for fat-loving toxins entering the body. Once deposited there, it is very difficult to remove them. Unless the excess fat is removed, they remain there with the possibility of being a continual source of toxicity.

TAP WATER

Your local tap water may contain unacceptable levels of fluoride, chlorine, or lead. You may need to install a water filter to decrease toxins that might be affecting your child.

BREAST FEEDING

Numerous studies confirm that breast-fed children enjoy better health than formula-fed infants. A study published in *Lancet* found that breast-fed children are more likely to score higher on IQ tests and less likely to have neurological dysfunction than formula-fed children. Another study compared nine-year old children who had been breast-fed to those that had been bottle-fed. These researchers found that the formula-fed children were twice as likely to have a neurological dysfunction that could contribute to behavioral and learning difficulties in school.

MENTAL/BEHAVIORAL TREATMENTS

COGNITIVE-BEHAVIORAL THERAPY

Cognitive-behavioral therapy helps people work on immediate issues. Rather than helping people understand their feelings and actions, it supports them directly in changing their behavior. The support might be practical assistance such as helping a child learn to think through tasks and organize their work. The support might be to encourage new behaviors by giving praise or rewards each time the child acts in the desired way. A cognitive-behavioral therapist might use such techniques to help a belligerent child learn to control his fighting or an impulsive teenager to think before she speaks.

RELAXATION

Try giving a child an herbal bath or foot soak. This is an excellent way of relaxing. Drink a tea made from one of the sedative herbs. Yoga exercises for children can help relax and center them. Also, use massage and acupressure; kids love to be touched.

SOCIAL SKILLS TRAINING

Your child can learn new behaviors. In social skills training, the therapist discusses and models appropriate behaviors like waiting for a turn, sharing toys, asking for help, or responding to teasing. Then the child is given a chance to practice. For example, a child might learn to "read" another person's facial expression and tone of voice, in order to respond more appropriately. Social skills training can help a child to learn how to join in group activities, make appropriate comments, and ask for help. A child might learn to see how his behavior affects others and develops new ways to respond when angry or pushed.

STRESS MANAGEMENT

Parents may also need to learn stress management methods, such as meditation, relaxation techniques, and exercise to increase their own tolerance to frustration, so that they can respond more calmly to their child's behavior.

SUPPORT GROUPS

These are groups that connect people who have common concerns. Many parents of children with ADD find it useful to join a local or national support group. These groups deal with issues concerning behavior disorders, and even ADD specifically. The national associations listed at the back of this book can explain how to contact a local chapter. Members of support groups share frustrations and successes, referrals to qualified specialists, and information about what works, as well as their hopes for themselves and their children. Sharing experiences with others who have similar problems help people know that they are not alone.

PSYCHOTHERAPY

Psychotherapy helps children with ADD to like and accept themselves despite their disorder. In psychotherapy, the child talks with the therapist about upsetting thoughts and feelings. They explore self-defeating patterns of behavior and learn alternative ways to handle their emotions. As they talk, the therapist tries to help them understand how changes could come about. If people dealing with ADD want to gain control of their symptomatic behaviors more directly, then they will need a more direct kind of intervention.

ALTERNATIVE HEALTH CARE

NATUROPATHIC HEALTH

Naturopathic medicine is founded on the healing power of nature. Within every person there is an innate ability for healing and maintaining health. The results of poor nutrition and lifestyle choices can lead to a decrease in resistance and the onset of disease. The symptoms of disease indicate improper functioning of organs and tissues. Bodies can be restored to normal function, effectively and naturally. This is possible with treatments that support and stimulate, rather than disrupt or suppress the body's innate ability to heal itself.

The holistic approach to health includes the physical, mental, emotional, and spiritual aspects of each individual. These aspects are inseparably connected to the well-being of the body. Therapies treat the whole person by supporting each of these areas throughout the healing process. The practice of naturopathic medicine prefers non-invasive treatments that minimize the risks of harmful side effects. Naturopathic treatment corrects the fundamental imbalances and restores proper function and health by safe, effective, and natural methods. Treatment includes showing ways to support the healing process and maintain renewed health. Our approach to health care can prevent minor illnesses from developing into more serious or chronic degenerative diseases.

Naturopathic physicians (N.D.) are educated and trained as primary-care providers. We are trained as general practitioners specializing in natural medicine. We treat a wide range of ailments and aim to restore health using an array of therapies that can include nutrition, herbal medicine, homeopathy, physical medicine (including hydrotherapy, exercise, and manipulation), natural childbirth, minor surgery, counseling techniques, and Oriental medicine. When you come to a naturopathic physician for your medical care, our objective is to determine the underlying cause of your condition or disease, whether it be of nutritional, lifestyle, mental, physicological, or environmental cause.

TRADITIONAL CHINESE MEDICINE

Traditional Chinese medicine views hyperactivity as the result of a "hot" liver. They have observed that a diet that is too acidic contributes to irritability and agitation in children. There is a tendency toward excitability when growth hormones are more active such as during periods of growth spurts. There are more irritations to a child's system when new teeth are coming in. Children who eat too many sweets tend to be restless at night. The Japanese call hyperactivity the "sweet bug" disease, and it is also associated with feeling itchy and restless.

Some doctors of Chinese medicine find that lightly touching the child is very helpful and effective during times of hyperactivity, and this includes before bedtime to help induce a better sleep. They also recommend cooling the liver fire with the Chinese herbal patent formula, Hsiao Yao Wan (bupleurum sedative pills). This famous Chinese patent remedy is widely available in herb stores.

Chapter 29

⊑

ARE DRUGS THE ANSWER?

Presently, there are about four million children taking Ritalin, or a similar drug, to control difficult behavioral conditions like ADD and hyperactivity. Onset of ADD usually occurs by the age of three, but diagnosis is generally after the child starts school. Something is seriously wrong when so many children must be "drugged" to control their behavior. No responsible person can feel comfortable about giving powerful drugs to children. Instead of treating a child with a drug first, a parent should try diet management and other alternatives like those suggested in this book. Children diagnosed with this disorder don't necessarily need drug treatment. It is essential that educational, psychological, social, as well as nutritional and dietary treatments be considered first. Allergies and metabolic dysfunctions also need to be considered.

"I'm very concerned that so many children are medicated so aggressively today for this disorder. Everything in my medical intuition tells me it's wrong. We do not have long-term studies on the effectiveness and safety of these drugs," says Dr. David Velkoff of the Drake Institute, in Los Angeles. A pediatrician and author of a book on hyperactivity, Dr. Ray Wunderlich, M.D., of St. Petersburg, Floida, advocates a more natural treatment to hyperactivity, and opposes treating children with drugs such as Ritalin. He believes it is almost never necessary.

Orthodox treatments use drugs to sedate and tranquilize children. This may remove some of the more obvious symptoms temporarily, but does nothing to deal with the cause. The parents are frequently told that nothing more can be done. The doctor may try to give some hope that the symptoms of hyperactive children will resolve themselves by the midteens. The Director of Princeton's Brain Bio Center, Carl C. Pfeiffer, Ph.D., M.D., writes that parents and physicians take the easy way out. His review of the medical literature suggests that long-time use of such drugs may result in brain damage, heart and artery disorders, and drug dependency. The drugs used can cause frequent and dangerous side effects. The use of psychoactive drugs in children should be a very serious step.

The more you study ADD, the less certain you are as to what it is, or whether it is a thousand different situations all called by the same name. This explains why almost all conventional physicians in the U.S. currently attempt to simply mask the child's symptoms with powerful drugs. One of the problems with the drug treatment of ADD is the frequent and dangerous side effects they produce. If you take your child off the drugs, what will you do? This affects not only your child's health, but the well-being of the whole family.

WHAT ARE THE MOST COMMON TYPES OF DRUGS?

It is important to understand the most commonly prescribed drugs for ADD. Much of this information is widely available in public medication publications such as the *Physician's Desk Reference* (PDR). Are you aware of the warnings, drug dependency risks, precautions, and adverse reactions related to their use? Don't depend on your physician to tell you about these drugs. You need to check out this information for yourself. The following is a summary of the drugs commonly used in the treatment of ADD.

PSYCHOSTIMULANTS

Psychostimulants include the following:

- Ritalin (Methylphenidate); also slow-release (SR) Ritalin
- Dexedrine (Dextroamphetamine)
- Cylert (Pemoline)
- Adderall (Obetrol)

The most commonly used drugs in the U.S. for children diagnosed with ADD are Ritalin and Dexedrine, both amphetamines. They are also known as "speed." These drugs have a calming effect and increase the attention span of some children. Stimulants may improve these children's sudden mood changes and ability to maintain attention, but numerous studies have failed to show improvement in retention of learning, overall achievement, or control of anger.

It helps to understand how these drugs work to calm hyperactive children. Stimulants increase the activity of neurotransmitters (brain chemicals) in parts of the brain that control the ability to pay attention and stay alert. They also seem to reduce distractibility, enhance concentration, and decrease motor restlessness and hyperactivity. It is often said that stimulants sedate children because their brains are somehow different from adults. This is not the case. Children respond to stimulants the same way adults do.

Major complaints of those taking Ritalin include irritability, nausea, appetite suppression, weight loss, insomnia or multiple varieties of sleep disturbances. Ten percent of patients on Ritalin complain of headaches. A physician must watch blood pressure and the pulse rate. Approximately 9 percent of children with attention deficit hyperactivity disorder treated with stimulant drugs develop tics and dyskinesias. Usually this is transient in nature, with less than one percent developing a chronic tic or Tourette's syndrome.

A more important issue in prescribing psychostimulants is the difficulty in achieving a therapeutic dose. Sometimes a person needs very little medication, others need much higher doses to sustain an effect. The most commonly made error in the treatment of ADD, especially with hyperactivity, is incorrect dosing.

TRYCYCLIC ANTIDEPRESSANTS

Trycyclic antidepressants (TCAs) are typically used to treat bedwetting and depression. They include:

- Tofranil or Janimine (Imipramine)
- Norpramin or Pertofane (Desipramine)
- Pamelor (Nortriptyline)

Tricyclic antidepressants exert their effect by acting upon norepinephrine and dopamine, the two major neurotransmitters in the attention system. They block the re-uptake of norepinephrine and dopamine, increasing the activity of these two chemicals in the brain. Tricyclics seem to have a different mechanism of action in ADD than they do in depression. It makes sense that the therapeutic dose range would also be different. In clinical practice a low dose seems to work best. While treatments with stimulants and tricyclics are extremely effective in enhancing concentration and attention, they often cannot sufficiently improve impulsivity, explosiveness, and irritability. Many conventional physicians just prescribe more drugs to deal with the additional symptoms.

Twenty to twenty-five percent of children with ADD do not show any response to stimulant drugs. These children are usually then given antidepressants. These drugs do not make a significant difference in delinquent behavior during adolescence, nor do short-term studies show positive changes in peer relations among children with ADD.

The majority of children with behavior problems show more improvement on Tofranil when it is given in low doses (five to ten milligrams per day). As experience with antidepressants accumulates, researchers and clinicians are aware that large doses may be useful in treating some forms of depression.

OTHER ANTIDEPRESSANTS

- Fluoxetine or Burproprion (these are MAOs)
- Wellbutrin (Bupropion) is unlike other tricylic antidepressants. It

tends to have a stimulating effect. It is currently popular among clinicians treating ADD. It is a potent dopamine re-uptake inhibitor.

- Mellaril (Thioridazine) is used to treat certain behavior problems in children
- Tegretol (Carbamazepine) is an anticonvulsant, a mood stabilizer, and used to treat aggressive behavior

A number of other agents, such as Fenfluramine, L-dopa and Amantadine, are being used to treat ADD. These are possibly useful drugs where others fail, but neither research nor clinical experience has shown these agents to be as effective as the psychostimulants and tricyclic antidepressants.

The truth is that 60-90 percent of students with ADD are treated with some form of drug medication. While these drugs can reduce children's hyperactive behavior temporarily, it does not solve the academic problems. Most studies show that drugs have few long-term benefits on academic achievement and social adjustment. Orthodox medicine has not achieved long-term success in treating hyperactivity. One study followed children with ADD into young adulthood. Regardless of the drug used, they failed more classes in high school and attended fewer colleges. Some research indicates that the effectiveness of stimulants for ADD may diminish over a period of months. Without using other tools and methods to help students with ADD, you are not really finding out the cause of your child's problems.

SPECIFIC DRUGS COMMONLY USED FOR TREATING ADD

ADDERALL (OBETROL)

Adderall is a psychostimulant that has been recently approved for the treatment of ADD. It is indicated for use in children three years of age and older. Adderall may improve attention span, decrease distractibility, and increase the ability to follow directions and finish tasks. This drug may also improve the patient's ability to think before acting (decrease impulsivity), decrease hyperactivity, and improve legibility of handwriting. In addition, aggression may decrease.

SIDE EFFECTS

The most frequently reported adverse reactions include anorexia, insomnia, stomach pain, headache, irritability, and weight loss. As with most psychostimulants, the possibility of growth suppression, motor tics, and Tourette's syndrome exists with Adderall treatment. In rare cases psychosis has been reported to get worse. Any psychostimulant has a high potential for abuse.

RITALIN (METHYLPHENIDATE HYDROCHLORIDE)

Ritalin is an amphetamine that works to slow children down. Unfortunately, too many psychiatrists believe the drug Ritalin is the answer to many behavioral problems, including ADD. Ritalin sales have increase over the past year more than 33 percent. About four million children receive Ritalin in the U.S. today.

The *Physician's Desk Reference* (PDR) warns not to give Ritalin to children under the age of six because safety and efficacy for this age group have not been established. They also caution that sufficient data on safety and efficacy of long-term use of Ritalin in children is not available.

Many parents who turn to Ritalin complain that their doctors do not discuss the number of harmful side effects associated with its use. One complaint filed against the British Columbia College of Physicians and Surgeons claimed the psychiatrist told the parents that Ritalin was "as safe as a vitamin." The British Columbia Chapter of the Citizen's Commission on Human Rights believes that Ritalin simply masks the real cause of ADD and is only being used because it is a quick fix.

SIDE EFFECTS

Side effects may include visual disturbances, the inability to fall or stay asleep, rapid heartbeat, nervousness, headaches, appetite loss resulting in weight loss, stomachaches, drowsiness, bed wetting, depression, liver toxicity and damage, facial tics, abnormal muscle movements, blood pressure changes, dizziness, and nausea. There are also rare reports of Tourette's syndrome, as well as toxic psychosis, anemia, and scalp hair loss.

Amphetamines, such as Ritalin, are appetite suppressants. They are used in weight loss or "diet" pills. Evidence shows that children on Ritalin consume less food and grow at a much slower rate. They usually catch up if they haven't been on the drug too long.

CAUTION

This drug should not be prescribed for anyone experiencing anxiety, tension and agitation, since the drug may aggravate these symptoms. It should not be prescribed for people with motor tics or Tourette's syndrome, or if there is a family history of these conditions. Do not use for normal fatigue, severe depression, or with a seizure disorder. Psychotic behavior can occur. Do not use machinery that requires you to be alert.

Excessive doses of Ritalin over a long period of time can produce addiction. It is possible to develop tolerance to this drug. This can make it necessary to take larger doses to produce the original effect. ADD can get much worse if you stop this drug suddenly. Severe depression as well as the effects of chronic over activity can surface during this time. Numerous suicides have occurred after drug withdrawal. Also, Ritalin may increase or decrease the effect of some drugs. The following drugs may need to have their doses adjusted when prescribed along with Ritalin:

• Anticonvulsants (Phenobarbital, Dilantin, Tegretol, and Primidone)
• Anti-inflammatories (Phenylbutazone)
• Tricyclic antidepressants (Tofranil and Norpramin)

OTHER INGREDIENTS PRESENT

Ritalin, depending on the dosage, may contain the dye D&C yellow No. 3 or 10, lactose, magnesium stearate, polyethylene glycol, starch, sucrose, and talc, as well as tragacanth, cetostearyl alcohol, mineral oil, povidone, and titanium dioxide.

Lately, Ritalin is being publicized as a drug that can "unlock" a child's potential. The view espoused by Ritalin promoters is that the drug works by correcting biochemical imbalances in the brain, but the plain truth is that no evidence exists that Ritalin makes any lasting change or that there is any brain imbalance to begin with. And there are no long-term studies on the safety and effectiveness of this drug. *Toxic Psychiatry* has recently stated that the long-term use of Ritalin causes irritability and hyperactivity. Ironically, these are the things that Ritalin is supposed to cure.

If a child does not respond to Ritalin, the next choice is usually Dexedrine. Ritalin and Dexedrine, while widely regarded as similar drugs, are not much alike at all. They have a different pharmacological profile, a different mechanism of action at the cellular level, and a not-so-subtle different effect on patients. The two drugs act upon separate neurotransmitter storage pools. Dexedrine is reported to be a "softer" drug than Ritalin. Ritalin sometimes makes patients feel as if their body is in overdrive. One patient described Dexedrine as a "caffeine-less" Ritalin. Most clinicians use Dexedrine as a second or third choice.

DEXEDRINE (DEXTROAMPHETAMINE SULFATE)

Amphetamines are appetite suppressants. Weight loss or diet pills contain similar compounds. Evidence shows that children on ten to fifteen milligrams of Dexedrine a day consume less food and gain weight at a much slower rate than children who discontinue this drug. They usually catch up in growth when the drug is discontinued, if they haven't waited too long.

Dexedrine is usually not given to children under three years old. Dexedrine is also a class II narcotic with the potential for dependency. The stimulant effect may give way to a let-down period of depression and fatigue. You can eventually become dependent on the drug and suffer from withdrawal symptoms when it is unavailable.

SIDE EFFECTS

Excessive restlessness, over stimulation, constipation, diarrhea, dizziness, dry mouth, headache, rapid heartbeat, sleeplessness, hives, exaggerated feeling of well-being or depression, sleeplessness, stomach and intestinal disturbances, tremors, uncontrollable twitching or jerking, unpleasant taste in the mouth, appetite suppression and weight loss, hyperactivity, personality changes, severe skin disease, schizophrenia-like thoughts and behavior are common to Dexedrine.

CAUTION

Your doctor should not prescribe Dexedrine if there is agitation, cardiovascular disease, glaucoma, hardening of the arteries, high blood pressure, or an overactive thyroid gland. Also, increasing the dosage of Dexedrine can lead to drug dependence. One of the inactive ingredients in Dexedrine is a yellow food coloring called tartrazine (FD&C Yellow No. 5). People who are sensitive to aspirin can have a severe allergic reaction to tartrazine. Dexedrine may impair judgment or coordination, and has been known to stunt a child's growth. Taking Dexedrine with certain foods or drugs can increase, decrease, or alter the effects. Antihistamines such as Benadryl can decrease the effect of Dexedrine.

CYLERT (PEMOLINE)

Cylert is a central nervous system stimulant. This is a class IV narcotic that does not usually cause dependency, but shouldn't be prescribed to children under the age of six.

SIDE EFFECTS

Insomnia, agitation, stomachaches, headaches, dizziness, drowsiness, hallucinations, loss of appetite, mild depression, nausea, seizures, skin rash, suppressed growth, abnormal movements, and abnormal liver functions tests. Recent research literature reports indicate that Cylert may precipitate attacks of Tourette's syndrome.

Caution

Safety and effectiveness of Cylert in children below the age of six years have not been established, as well as the long-term effect in children. Warn your child to be careful climbing stairs or participating in activities that require mental alertness if they are on Cylert. The administration of Cylert may make symptoms of behavior disturbance and thought disorder worse. Administer with caution to anyone with significantly impaired kidney function. Perform liver function tests prior to and periodically during therapy. Discontinue the use of Cylert if there are abnormalities found on the test.

Cylert generally does not induce as dramatic results as Ritalin or Dexedrine. Although there have been no reports that Cylert is physically addictive, it is chemically similar to a same class of drugs that are potentially addictive. Psychotic children may experience increasingly disordered thoughts and behavioral disturbances. Taking Cylert with other drugs can increase, decrease, or alter the effects.

NORPRAMIN (DESIPRAMINE HYDROCHLORIDE)

Norpramin is a tricylic antidepressant used in the treatment of depression and ADD. The positive effects may take up to three weeks before they are apparent.

Side Effects

Dry mouth, decreased appetite, headache, dizziness, constipation, diarrhea, mild tachycardia, anxiety, abdominal cramps, urinary problems, fatigue, high or low blood pressure, hives, inflammation of the mouth, insomnia, lack of coordination, breast enlargement, and disorientation are common to this drug. Check the *Physicians Desk Reference* (PDR) for more examples of side effects.

CAUTION

Serious reactions can occurr when Norpramin is taken with another type of antidepressant. Discontinue Norpramin gradually because of the side effects. Before using Norpramin, let your doctor know there is heart or thyroid disease, or a seizure disorder. This drug can affect your child's ability to stay alert and increase the skin's sensitivity to sunlight.

If Norpramin is taken with certain other drugs, the effects of either could be increased, decreased, or altered. These drugs include: Cimetidine (Tagamet), Proventil, Bentyl, fluoxetine (Prozac), Guanethidine (Ismelin) Halcion, Valium, and thyroid medications (Synthroid).

Starting in 1990, the package insert for the Merrell Dow Pharmaceutical brand of Norpramin included the following statement in the Adverse Reactions section, "There has been a report of an 'acute collapse' and 'sudden death' in an eight-year-old male, treated for two years for hyperactivity. There have been additional reports of sudden death in children."

TOFRANIL (IMIPRAMINE HYDROCHLORIDE)

Tofranil is a tricyclic antidepressant used to treat depression. It is also used to treat bedwetting in children age six and older. Some doctors prescribe Tofranil to treat attention deficit disorder in children.

SIDE EFFECTS

Cough, high or low blood sugar, hives, insomnia, intestinal blockage, lack of coordination, nightmares, odd taste in mouth, skin itching and rash, sore throat, sweating, dry mouth, decreased appetite, headache, stomachache and other intestinal disorders, dizziness, constipation, and irregular heart beat are common to Tofranil. Check the PDR for additional side effects.

CAUTION

Check for any pre-existing cardiac defects before starting this drug. Discontinue gradually. There are reports of serious reactions when these types of drugs are combined with MAO inhibitors. Tofranil can interact with certain other drugs. The effect could be increased, decreased, or altered. It is a long list so consult your PDR for more information.

WELLBUTRIN (BUPROPION HYDROCHLORIDE)

Wellbutrin is an antidepressant. Some of the symptoms this drug is used for are changes in sleep, psychomotor agitation, loss of interest in usual activities, increased fatigue, feelings of guilt or worthlessness, slowed thinking or impaired concentration.

SIDE EFFECTS

Edema, nonspecific rashes, thirst, liver damage, wetting at night, urinary incontinence during the day, uncoordination, seizures, depression, flu-like symptoms, aches and pains, dream abnormalities, ringing in the ears, agitation, dry mouth, headaches or migraines, constipation, and tremors. There may also be abnormalities in mental status, gastrointestinal disturbances, nausea and vomiting, and sleep disturbances. Ten percent of the people tested initially had enough side effects to discontinue this drug.

A substantial amount of people treated with Wellbutrin experience some degree of increased restlessness, agitation, anxiety, and insomnia, especially shortly after the initiation of treatment. Other side effects included delusions, hallucinations, and confusion. Altered appetite and weight loss of greater than five pounds occurred in 28 percent of Wellbutrin patients. It may impair their ability to perform tasks requiring judgment, motor or cognitive skills. There may be an increase in locomotor activity. Wellbutrin is associated with seizures in approximately 4 out of 1000 patients treated at doses up to 450 milligrams a day. This incidence of seizures may exceed other antidepressants by as much as fourfold.

Caution

The toxicity of this drug is not known, especially in long-term use. In animal studies there was an increase in incidence of liver problems as well as liver injury. The child needs to be closely monitored for toxic effects. The safety and effectiveness of Wellbutrin in individuals under eighteen years old have not been established. The PDR does not show any dosage for the administration of this drug in the use with children, yet it is being prescribed for them. This drug can change the effects of other drugs taken at the same time.

DRUGS SHOULD BE THE LAST RESOURCE

Simply stated, drugs are not a satisfactory treatment for many children with ADD or hyperactivity. Some children do not respond to these drugs and sometimes suffer disturbing side effects. Even if children respond well to drugs, some parents are uncomfortable having their child medicated. These drugs may only work for part of the day or cause a rebound effect making symptoms even worse. Many of the most popular drugs treat the symptoms of distractibility and hyperactivity, but other behavior problems may not be addressed.

Although these drugs, when prescribed appropriately, may be effective in controlling behavior problems, they do not treat the cause. Reserve drugs as a last effort, after all other possibilities have been ruled out. It does take some time to find the cause of ADD rather than mask it with drugs. Drugs should never be the only treatment your child receives. I question the quick-fix mentality that can make Ritalin-type drugs the cornerstone of treatment for ADD. Unfortunately, people may see immediate improvement from the drugs and think this type of medication is all that is needed.

Children may pay better attention and complete their work with some of these drugs, but they cannot increase knowledge or improve poor social skills. The drugs alone do not help children feel better about themselves or cope with problems. They also do not replace family therapy, special education, or other treatments. Part of the problem is the insurance companies. They will pay for your visit if it is conventional medicine, but often will not cover preventive and natural treatments.

Parents need to be clear about the benefits and potential risks of using these drugs. Is Ritalin, or any other drug, prescribed unnecessarily? Children on drugs should have regular checkups. Parents should also talk regularly with the child's teachers and doctor about how the child is doing. This is especially important when a drug is first started, restarted, or when changing the dosage. Doctors should carefully weigh the potential side effects against the benefits before prescribing drugs.

Critics argue that many children who do not have a true attention disorder are medicated as a way to control their disruptive behaviors. Is your child one of these? Even if your child responds well to a stimulant drug, it doesn't mean they have ADD. Stimulants allow many people to focus and pay better attention. The improvement is just more noticeable in children with ADD.

Resource Guide

Products for the Allergic Person

Bob's Red Mill Natural Foods, Inc., 5209 SE International Way, Milwaukie, OR 97222. (800) 553-2258 or in Oregon call (503) 654-3215. Send for a catalog. Bob's Red Mill not only mills, manufactures, and distributes whole-grain natural foods, but they also sell bread mixes for bread machines and a fat replacer for all baked goods. They also offer a wide selection of books on beans, grains, flours, and gluten-free and wheat-free cooking and baking.

Dietary Specialties, PO Box 227, Rochester, NY 14601. (716) 263-2787. Offers a wide selection of pre-packaged gluten-free muffins, cookies, and bread mixes.

Ener-G Foods, Inc., 5960 1st Ave S, Seattle, WA, 98124. (800) 331-5222 or in Washington call (206) 767-6660. Write for a list of alternative food products including gluten-free and wheat-free foods; catalog available.

The Green Earth, 2545 Prairie Ave, Evanston, IL 60201. (708) 475-0205. A source of organic natural foods, nuts, dried fruits, meats and poultry.

National Coalition Against Misuse of Pesticides, 530 Seventh St, Washington, DC 20003. (202) 543-5450. More information about organic foods.

Peaceful Valley Farm Supply, PO Box 220, Grass Valley, CA 95945. (916) 272-4769. Organic gardening supplies; catalog available.

Special Foods, 9207 Shotgun Court, Springfield, VA 22150. (703) 644-0991. Offers unusual bread, flours, and infant formulas that are milk and gluten free.

Spectrum Naturals of Petaluma, California. Manufacturer of *Spectrum Spread,* a non-hydrogenated, non-dairy spread. It is available in natural-foods stores nationwide.

Food & Environmental Allergy Network, 4744 Holly Avenue, Fairfax, VA 22030. (703) 691-3179. Parents seeking advice on how to handle children with food allergies can send a stamped, self-addressed envelope to this network.

Food and Drug Administration (FDA), Parklawn Bldg, 5600 Fisher's Ln, # 14-71, Rockville, MD 20857. Attn: Commissioner. Write to the FDA

Commissioner with your concerns about foods and drugs.

The Natural Grocer Radio Show. Features expert guests discussing all aspects of alternative health and natural healing. The show is now heard weekly in Phoenix, AZ, on KRDS 1190 AM, Saturday 12- 1:30 p.m; in Miami/Ft. Lauderdale, FL, on WWNN 980 AM, Monday-Friday 3-4 p.m; in Chicago, IL, on WYLL 106.7 FM Saturday 12-1 p.m; in Los Angeles, CA, on KRBT 740 AM, Saturday 12:30-1:30 p.m.

Practical Allergy Research Foundation, PO Box 60, Buffalo, NY 14223-0060. (726) 875-0398. Books, audio tapes and educational videos for the public and physicians on environmental-related health and emotional illnesses in children. Doris Rapp, MD, founder of the foundation, has compiled a comprehensive library on environmental illness and its impact on children. They also offer her best-selling book *Is This Your Child?*

Preconception Care Foundation, 5724 Clymer Road, Quakertown, PA 18951. A guidebook for preconception care is being prepared and should be available.

Well Mind Association, 4649 Sunnyside North, Seattle, WA 98103. (206) 547-6167. A non-profit organization dedicated to helping victims of brain dysfunction and environmental sensitivities. They publish a newsletter and have a resource library.

Organic foods by mail! You can bring organic farmers' products to your doorstep year-round. Mail-order organic foods often come directly from the producers and may be fresher than supermarket foods. Most of the growers sell in bulk. These sources are from *Green Groceries: A Mail Order Guide to Organic Foods* (Harper Collins, 1992). If you live in an area that encourages and promotes organic foods, get to know your local organic growers and businesses. If you don't live close to organic products, the following mail-order companies may be more convenient. They sell organic produce and products in many categories. This offers you a one-stop shopping advantage:

Allergy Resources, Inc.
195 Huntington Beach Dr
Colorado Springs, CO 80921
(719) 488-3630

Rising Sun Organic Food
PO. Box 627, PA 150 & I-80
Milesburg, PA 16853
(814) 355-9850

Walnut Acres Organic Farms
Walnut Acres Rd
Penns Creek, PA 17862
(800) 433-3998

The Green Earth
2545 Prairie Ave
Evanston, IL 60201
(800) 322-3662

The following companies sell organic specialty items. Their individual specialty will be noted after their address. Most companies offer free catalogs:

Starr Organic Produce
P.O. Box 561502
Miami, FL 33256-1502
(305) 262-1242
Organically grown tropical
fruits as well as dried fruit

Diamond Organics
P.O. Box 2159
Freedom, CA 95019
(800) 922-2396
Organic varieties of lettuce,
fresh herbs, vegies, fruit

Morningland Dairy
Rt. 1, Box 188B
Mt. View, MO 65548
Organic raw milk and
cheeses

D'Artagnan
399-419 St. Paul Ave.
Jersey City, NJ 07306
(800) DAR-TAGN
Organic meat and poultry

Windy River Farm
P.O Box 312
Merlin, OR 97532
(503) 476-8979
Organic culinary herbs, dried
fruits, vegetables

Eagle Organic/Natural Food
407 Church Ave.
Huntsville, AR 72703
(501) 738-2203
Organic whole-grain flour,
cereals, mixex, beans, coffee

Community Mill & Bean
267 RT 89 South
Savannah, NY 13146
(800) 755-0554
Organic baking mixes, whole grains, beans.

Community-supported agriculture (CSA) is an idea developed about twenty-five years ago in Europe. CSA is a way for each of us to become directly involved in the food system that nourishes us. This program gives people a direct connection to organic farmers. It provides high-quality food at a reasonable price by establishing a direct link between those who grow food and those who eat it.

The individuals and families who associate with a CSA farm pledge to support it annually. This is done by buying shares in the harvest at the beginning of each year. The income from these shares covers the operating expenses of the farm. In return, the farm provides the shareholders with fresh food throughout the season. Some CSA farm shareholders can work on the farm a few hours during the season as part of their support.

CSA farms have certified organically grown crops. They are dedicated to preserving the health of the soil, to ecological balance, and diversity. Goals are to rediscover, develop, and use sustainable methods and practices for growing a variety of nutritious and healthful foods for local consumption. The farmers strive to restore and maintain the vitality of the earth through the use of composts, cover cropping, crop rotation, and natural methods of fertilization, disease and pest control. Look for a CSA farm in your area, and become a shareholder.

SUPPORT GROUPS AND ORGANIZATIONS

ADD Warehouse, 300 NW 70th Avenue, Plantation, FL 33317 (800) 233-9273 (US only), Phone (305) 792-8944, Fax (305) 792-8545. Distributes books, tapes, videos, assessment on attention deficit hyperactivity disorders. A central location for ordering many of the books listed above. Call for catalog.

Attention Deficit Information Network (Ad-IN), 475 Hillside Avenue, Needham, MA 02194, (617) 455-9895. Provides up-to-date information on current research, regional meetings. Aids in finding solutions to practical problems faced by adults and children with an attention disorder.

Center for Mental Health Services, Office of Consumer, Family, and Public Information, 5600 Fishers Lane, Room 15-105, Rockville, MD 20857, (301) 443-2792. This national center, a component of the U.S. Public HealthService, provides a range of information on mental health, treatment, and support services.

Children and Adults with Attention Deficit Disorders (CH.A.D.D.), 499 NW 70th Avenue, Suite 109, Plantation, FL 33317, (954) 587-3700, Fax (954) 587-4599. A major advocate and key information source for people dealing with attention disorders. Sponsors support groups and publishes two newsletters concerning attention disorders for parents and professionals. CH.A.D.D. has become the national organization for children and adults with ADD. They work at influencing public policy, sponsor the major ADD conferences, and provide support to parents of children with ADD through local chapters. (Note: I find it distressing, as well as a sign of gross ignorance, that the national CH.A.D.D. group readily suggests medications such as psychostimulants without any endorsement of any alternative and natural treatments. Their medical position mentions only the use of drugs. They say they support public and professional education, but they obviously have not fully investigated the progress that many children are making with alternative treatments.)

Council for Exceptional Children, 11920 Association Drive, Reston, VA 22091, (703) 620-3660. Provides publications for educators. Can also provide referral to ERIC (Educational Resource Information Center) and Clearinghouse for Handicapped and Gifted Children.

Federation of Families for Children's Mental Health, 1021 Prince Street, Alexandria, VA 22314, (703) 684-7710. Provides information, support, and referrals through federation chapters throughout the country. This national parent-run organization focuses on the needs of children with broad mental health problems.

Feingold Association of the United States, Box 6550, Alexandria, VA 22306. (800) 321-3287 or (516) 369-9340. This group offers a natural dietary approach with a food list, handbook, and a newsletter. They hope to educate about the necessity of eliminating synthetic colors, preservative from the diet, and the possibility of hidden food allergies.The overall goal is to enhance parent's ability to do these natural therapies at home. As support they offer contact with a network of other parents dealing with this issue.

HEATH Resource Center, American Council on Education, 1 Dupont Circle, Suite 800,Washington, DC 20036. (800) 544-3284. A national clearinghouse on post-high school education for people with disabilities.

NAMI Helpline. (800) 950-6264 for information about contacting your state and local affiliates. NAMI Office (703) 524-7600, Fax (703) 524-9094, Internet at NAMIofc@aol.com. The NAMI Helpline can assist with questions and requests for material. A series of brochures are also provided.

National Association of Private Schools for Exceptional Children, 1522 K Street, NW, Suite 1032,Washington, DC 20005, (202) 408-3338. Provides referrals to private special education programs.

National Attention Deficit Disorder Association (NADDA), (800) 487-2282

National Clearinghouse for Alcohol and Drug Information, PO Box 2345, Rockville, MD 20847, (800) 729-6686. Provides information on the risks of alcohol during pregnancy, and fetal alcohol syndrome.

Optometric Extension Program Foundation, Inc., 1921 E. Carnegie Ave. Suite. 3-L, Santa Ana, CA 92705-5510 or phone (714) 250-8070 or fax (714) 250-8157.

Parents Active for Vision Education (P.A.V.E.), 7331 Hamlet Avenue, San Diego, CA 92120-1923 or phone (619) 464-0687 or fax (619) 582-6109. This is a non-profit resource and support organization whose mission is to raise public awareness of the crucial relationship between vision and achievement. It was founded by parents and teachers who had children suffered the effects of undiagnosed vision problems.

Sibling Information Network, A.J. Pappanikou Center, 1776 Ellington Road,

South Windsor, CT 06074, (860) 648-1205. Publishes a newsletter for and about siblings of children with special needs.

Touch and Movement. For information on the effects contact Oregon Hope and Help Center, Inc., 152 Arthur St., P.O. Box 406, Woodburn, OR 97071, (503-981-0635).

Tourette's Syndrome Association, 42-40 Bell Boulevard, Bayside, NY 11361. (718) 224-2999. State and local chapters provide national information, advocacy, research, and support.

BIBLIOGRAPHY

JOURNALS

Abikoff H, Courtney M, Pelham WE Jr, Koplewicz HS: *Teachers: Ratings of Disruptive Berhaviors: The Influence of Halo Effects.* Journal of Abnormal Child Psychology 1993; 21(5):519-33.

Alston CY, Romney DM: *A Comparison of Medicated and Nonmedicated ADHD Boys.* Acta Paedopsychiatrica 1992;55(2):65-70.

Anastopoulos AD, Guevremont DC, Shelton TL, DuPaul GJ: *Parenting Stress Among Families of Children with Attention Deficit Hyperactivity Disorder.* Journal of Abnormal Child Psychology 1992;20(5):503-20.

Anastopoulos AD, DuPaul GJ, Barkley RA: *Stimulant Medication and Parent Training Therapies for Attention Deficit-Hyperactivity Disorder* (Review). Journal of Learning Disabilities 1991;24(4):210-8.

Atkins MS, Pelham WE: *School-Based Assessment of Attention Deficit Hyperactivity Disorder* (Review). Journal of Learning Disabilities 1991;24(4):197-204, 255.

Balthazor MJ, Wagner RK, Pelham WE: *The Specificity of the Effects of Stimulant Medication on Classroom Learning-Related Measures of Cognitive Processing for Attention Deficit Disorder Children.* Journal of Abnormal Child Psychology 1991;19(1):35-52.

Barkely R: *A Review of Stimulant Drug Research with Hyperactive Children.* Journal of Child Psychology and Psychiatry 1977;18:137-165.

Bellak L, Stanley RK, Lewis AO: *Attention Deficit Disorder Psychosis as a Diagnostic Category.* Psychiatric Developments 1987;3:239-262.

Biederman J, Faraone SV, Milberger S, Doyle A: *Diagnosis of Attention Deficit Hyperactivity Disorder from Parent Reports Predict Diagnosis Based on Teacher Reports.* Journal of the American Academy of Child & Adolescent Psychiatry 1993;32(2):315-7.

Biederman J, Faraone SV, Keenan K, Tsuang MT: *Evidence of Familial Association Between Attention Deficit Disorder and Major Affective Disorders.* Archives of General Psychiatry 1991;48(7):633-42.

Biederman J, Faraone SV, Mick E, Spencer T, Wilens T, Kiely K, Guite J, Ablon JS, Reed E, Warburton R: *High Risk for Attention Deficit Hyperactivity Disorder Among Children of Parents with Childhood Onset of the Disorder.* American Journal of Psychiatry 1995; 152(3):431-5.

Bloomquist ML, August GJ, Ostrander R: *Effects of a School-Based Cognitive-*

Behavioral Intervention for ADHD Children. Journal of Abnormal Child Psychology 1991;19(5):591-605.

Colgan M, Colgan L, *Do nutrient supplements and dietary changes affect learning and emotional reactions of children with learning difficulties? A controlled series of 16 cases.* Nutrition and Health 1984;3:69-77.

Collipp, PJ: *Manganese in infant formulas and learning disability.* Annuals Nutrition Metabolism 1983;9183; 27:488-94.

Cantwell DP, Baker L: *Association Between Attention Deficit-Hyperactivity and Learning Disorders* (Review). Journal of Learning Disabilities 1991;24(2):88-95.

David, OJ: *Association Between Lower Level Lead Concentrations and Hyperactivity in Children.* Environmental Health Perspectives 1974;17-25.

Derrick, Lonsdale, MD: *Criminal Behavior and Nutrition.* Journal of Advancement in Medicine, Summer 1992;5(2):115-123.

DiBattista D, Shepherd ML: *Primary School Teachers' Beliefs and Advice to Parents Concerning Sugar Consumption and Activity in Children.* Psychological Reports 1993; 72(1):47-55.

Dykman RA, Ackerman PT: *Attention Deficit Disorder and Specific Reading Disability: Separate but Often Overlapping Disorders.* Journal of Learning Disabilities 1991;24(2):96-103.

Egger J, Stolla A, McEwen LM: *Controlled Trial of Hyposensitization in Children with Food-Induced Hyperkinetic Syndrome.* Lancet 1992;339(8802):1150-3.

Egger, Joseph: *Controlled Trial of Hyposensitization in Children with Food-Induced Hyperkinetic Syndrome,* The Lancet, May 1992:339:1150-1153.

Egger J, Carter CM, Graham PJ, Gumley D, Soothill JF: *Controlled Trial of Oliogantigenic Treatment in the Hyperkinetic Syndrome.* The Lancet 1985;i:540-5.

Elia J, Gulotta C, Rose SR, Marin G, Rapoport JL: *Thyroid Function and Attention Deficit Hyperactivity Disorder.* Journal of the American Academy of Child & Adolescent Psychiatry 1994;33(2):169-72.

Epstein MA, Shaywitz SE, Shaywitz BA, Woolston JL: *The Boundaries of Attention Deficit Disorder.* Journal of Learning Disabilities 1991;24(2):78-86.

Fehlings DL, Roberts W, Humphries T, Dawe G: *Attention Deficit Hyperactivity Disorder: Does Cognitive Behavioral Therapy Improve Home Behavior?* Journal of Developmental & Behavioral Pediatrics 1991;12(4):223-8.

Forehand R, Wierson M, Frame C, Kempton T, Armistead L: *Juvenile Delinquency Entry and Persistence: Do Attention Problems Contribute to Conduct Problems?* Journal of Behavior Therapy & Experimental

Psychiatry 1991;22(4):261-4.

Forness SR, Cantwell DP, Swanson JM, Hanna GL, Youpa D: *Differential Effects of Stimulant Medication on Reading Performance of Boys with Hyperactivity with and without Conduct Disorder.* Journal of Learning Disabilities 1991;24(5):304-10.

Gans DA: *Sucrose and Delinquent Behavior: Coincidence or Consequence?* (Review). Critical Reviews in Food Science & Nutrition 1991;30(1):23-48.

Giddan JJ: *Communication Issues in Attention Deficit Hyperactivity Disorder.* Child Psychiatry & Human Development 1991;22(1):45-51.

Golden GS: *Role of Attention Deficit Hyperactivity Disorder in Learning Disabilities* (Review). Seminars in Neurology 1991;11(1):35-41.

Gross-Tsur V, Shalev RS, Amir N: *Attention Deficit Disorder: Association with Familial-Genetic Factors.* Pediatric Neurology 1991;7(4):258-61.

Hedges, Harold H, MD: *The Elimination Diet as a Diagnostic Tool.* AFP Journal, Nov 1992;46(5):77S-85S.

Horn WF, Ialongo NS, Pascoe JM, Greenberg G, Packard T, Lopez M, Wagner A, Puttler L: *Additive Effects of Psychostimulants, Parent Training, and Self-Control Therapy with ADHD Children.* Journal of the American Academy of Child & Adolescent Psychiatry 1991;30(2):233-40.

Huessy H: *Medication vs Behavioral Management.* American Journal of Orthopsychiatry 1989; 59:153-155.

Hughes, EC, *Case Report: A Chemically Defined Diet in Diagnosis and Management of Food Sensitivity in Minimal Brain Dysfunction,* Annals of Allergy, March, 1979;174-176.

Hynd GW, Lorys AR, Semrud-Clikeman M, Nieves N, Huettner MI, Lahey BB: *Attention Deficit Disorder without Hyperactivity: A Distinct Behavioral and Neurocognitive Syndrome.* Journal of Child Neurology 1991;6 Suppl:S37-43.

Jensen PS, Shervette RE 3d, Xenakis SN, Richters J: *Anxiety and Depressive Disorders in Attention Deficit Disorder with Hyperactivity: New Findings.* American Journal of Psychiatry 1993;150(8):1203-9.

Kaplan, BJ, McNicol J, Conte RA, and Moghadam, HK. *Dietary Replacement in Preschool-aged Hyperactive Boys.* Pediatrics 1989;83(1):7-17.

Kasten EF, Coury DL, Heron TE: *Educator's Knowledge and Attitudes Regarding Stimulants in the Treatment of ADHD.* Journal of Developmental & Behavioral Pediatrics 1992; 13(3):215-9.

Kelly DP, Aylward GP: *Attention Deficits in School-Aged Children and Adolescents: Current Issues and Practice* (Review). Pediatric Clinics of North America 1992;39(3):487-512.

Kelly DP, Kelly BJ, Jones ML, Moulton NJ, Verhulst SJ, Bell SA: *Attention*

Deficits in Children and Adolescents with Hearing Loss. A Survey. American Journal of Diseases of Children 1993;147(7):737-41.

Langseth L, Dowd J: *GlucoseTolerance and Hyperkinesis,* Fd.Cosmet.Toxicol 1978;16:129.

Lee SW: *Biofeedback as a Treatment for Childhood Hyperactivity: A Critical Review of the Literature* (Review). Psychological Reports 1991;68(1):163-92.

Levinson HN: *Dramatic Favorable Responses of Children with Learning Disabilities or Dyslexia and ADD to Anti-motion Sickness Medications.* Perceptual & Motor Skills 1991;73(3 Pt 1):723-38.

Levy F: *The Dopamine Theory of Attention Deficit Hyperactivity Disorder* (Review). Australian & New Zealand Journal of Psychiatry 1991;25(2):277-83.

Linden M, Habib T, Radojevic V: *A controlled study of EEG biofeedback effects on cognitive and behavioral measures with attention-deficit disorder and learning-disabled children.* Biofeedback & Self-Regulation 1993;18:142-143.

Lubar JF: *Discourse on the development of EEG Diagnostics and Biofeedback for Attention Deficit/Hyperactivity Disorders* (Review). Biofeedback & Self Regulation 1991;16(3):201-25.

Mantzicopoulos PY, Morrison D: *A Comparison of Boys and Girls with Attention Problems: Kindergarten Through Second Grade.* American Journal of Orthopsychiatry 1994; 64(4):522-33.

Margalit M, Almougy K: *Classroom Behavior and Family Climate in Students with Learning Disabilities and Hyperactive Behavior.* Journal of Learning Disabilities 1991;24(7):406-12.

McGee R, Stanton WR, Sears MR: *Allergic Disorders and Attention Deficit Disorder in Children.* Journal of Abnormal Child Psychology 1993;21(1):79-88.

McGee R, Williams S, Feehan M: *Attention Deficit Disorder and Age of Onset of Problem Behaviors.* Journal of Abnormal Child Psychology 1992;20(5):487-502.

Minder B, Das-Smaal EA, Brand EF, Orlebeke JF: *Exposure to Lead and Specific Attention Problems in School Children.* Journal of Learning Disabilities 1994;27(6):393-9.

O'Brien, M: *Attention Deficit Disorder with Hyperactivity. A Review.* Journal of Special Education 1986;20(3), 281-297.

O'Shea, JA, and Porter, S.F.: *Double-Blind Study Reconfirms Link Between Allergens and Some Hyperkinetics.* Journal of Learning Disabilities 1988;vol.14:189-91.

Ouellette EM: *Legal Issues in the Treatment of Children with Attention Deficit*

Hyperactivity Disorder (Review). Journal of Child Neurology 1991;6 Suppl:S68-75.

Perkin, JE: *Maternal Influences on the Development of Food Allergy in the Infant.* Food Allergies in Infants 1990;5(4):6-34.

Pihl, Robert O, PhD, and Peterson, Jordan B, PhD: *Attention Deficit Hyperactivity Disorder, Childhood Conduct Disorder and Alcoholism - Is There An Association?* Alcohol, Health and Research World 1991;15(1):25-31.

Pisterman S, Firestone P, McGrath P, Goodman JT, Webster I, Mallory R, Goffin B: *The Role of Parent Training in Treatment of Preschoolers with ADDH.* American Journal of Orthopsychiatry 1992;62(3):397-408.

Pollitt, E, Leibel R: *Iron Deficiency Anemia and Scholastic Achievement in Young Adolescents.* Journal of Pediatrics 1976;88:372-81.

Potashkin BD, Bedkles N: *Relative Efficacy of Ritalin and Biofeedback Treatments in the Management of Hyperactivity.* Biof Self Reg Dec 1990;15(4):305-15.

Riccio CA, Hynd GW, Cohen MJ, Hall J, Molt L: *Comorbidity of Central Auditory Processing Disorder and Attention Deficit Hyperactivity Disorder.* Journal of the American Academy of Child & Adolescent Psychiatry 1994;33(6):849-57.

Rowe, KS and Rowe, KJ: *Synthetic Food Coloring and Behavior; A Dose Response Effect in a Double-Blind, Placebo-Controlled, Repeated Measures Study.* Journal of Pediatrics 1994; 125:691-8.

Schoenthaler, Stephen J, PhD: *Applied Nutrition and Behavior,* Journal of Applied Nutrition 1990; 43(1):31-39.

Sciarillo, William G, ScD: *Lead Exposure and Child Behavior.* American Journal of Public Health 1992;82(10):1356-1359.

Sharma V, Halperin JH, Newcorn JN, Wolf LE: *The Dimension of Focused Attention: Relationship to Behavior and Cognitive Functioning in Chidlren.* Perceptual & Motor Skills 1991;72(3 Pt 1):787-93.

Shouse, MN, Lubar, JF: *Operant Conditioning of EEG Rhythms and Ritalin in the Treatment of Hyperkinesis.* Biofeedback & Self-Regulation 1979; 4(4)(:301-312.

Stein, MA: *Attention Deficit-Hyperactivity Disorde.* The New England Journal of Medicine 1993;329(13):966.

Sterman, MB, MacDonald, LR: *Effects of central cortical EEG feedback training on seizure incidence in poorly controlled epileptics.* Epilepsia 1978;19:207-222

Swanson JM, Cantwell D, Lerner M, McBurnett K, Hanna G: *Effects of*

Stimulant Medication on Learning in Children with ADHD (Review). Journal of Learning Disabilities 1991;24(4):219-30,255.

Swanson JM, Posner M, Potkin S, Bonforte S, Youpa D, Fiore C, Cantwell D, Crinella F: *Activating Tasks for the Study of Visual-Spatial Attention in ADHD Children: A Cognitive Anatomic Approach* (Review). Journal of Child Neurology 1991;6 Suppl:S119-27.

Voeller KK: *Clinical Management of Attention Deficit Hyperactivity Disorder* (Review). Journal of Child Neurology 1991;6 Suppl:S51-67.

Wacker Foundation: *Mother's Milk Increases IQ, Reduces Neurological Problems.* Crime Times 1996, Vol 2, No 1. (Dept. 132, 1106 North Gilbert Rd, Suite 2, Mesa, Arizona 85203)

Weitzman, Michael, MD: *Maternal Smoking and Behavior Problems of Children.* Pediatrics, Sept 1992;90(3);342-349.

Weinberg WA, Emslie GJ: *Attention Deficit Hyperactivity Disorder: The Differential Diagnosis.* (Review). Journal of Child Neurology 1991;6 Suppl:S23-36.

Weiss RE, Stein MA, Trommer B, Refetoff S: *Attention Deficit Hyperactivity Disorder and Thyroid Function.* Journal of Pediatrics 1993;123(4):539-45.

Whalen CK, Henker B: *Therapies for Hyperactive Children: Comparisons, Combinations, and Compromises* (Review). Journal of Consulting & Clinical Psychology 1991; 59(1):126-37.

Whalen CK, Henker B: *Social Impact of Stimulant Treatment for Hyperactive Children.* Journal of Learning Disabilities 1991;24(4):231-41.

Zelko FA: *Comparison of Parent-Completed Behavior Rating Scales: Differentiating Boys with ADD from Psychiatric and Normal Controls.* Journal of Developmental & Behavioral Pediatrics 1991;12(1):31-7.

BOOKS

Austin, Phylis; Agatha Thrash, MD; Calvin Thrash, MD. *More Natural Remedies—What to do to Prevewnt and Treat Disease...Naturally.* Thrash Publication, Seale, Al, 1983.

Balch, James F, MD, Phyllis A Balch, CNC. *Prescription for Nutritional Healing.* Avery Publishing Group, NY, 1990.

Ballentine, Rudolph, MD. *Diet & Nutrition - A Holistic Approach.* The Himalayan International Institute, Honedale, PA, 1978.

Barnes, Broda, MD. *Hypothyroidism: The Unsuspected Illness.* Fitzhenry & Whiteside Ltd., Toronto, 1976.

Bauman, Edward; Brint, Armand; Piper, Lorin; Wright, Pamela. *The Holistic Health Handbook.* And/Or Press, Berkeley, CA, 1978.

Bricklin, Mark. *The Practical Encyclopedia of Natural Healing.* Rodale Press, NY, 1983.

Brody, Jane E. *Jane Brody's Nutrition Book.* W.W. Norton & Co, NY, 1981.

Buechler, Lynn H; Lawrence D. Chilnick; Janet S. Chilnick; Jayne Jacobson; Regina C. Vengrow; Theresa Waldron. *The PDR Pocket Guide to Prescription Drugs.* Pocket Books, NY, NY, 1996.

Dadd, Debra L. *The Nontoxic Home & Office.* GP Putnam's Sons, NY, NY, 1992.

Dean, Ward, MD, Morgenthaler, John. *Smart Drugs& Nutrients - How To Improve Your Memory and Increase Your Intelligence Using the Latest Discoveries in Neuroscience.* Health Freedom Pub, 1990.

Elkins, Rita. *Depression and Natural Medicine.* Woodland Publishing, Pleasant Grove, UT, 1995.

Elkins, Rita. *The Complete Home Health Advisor.* Woodland Publishing, Pleasant Grove, UT, 1995.

Frompovich, Catherine, DSc, ND. *Understanding Body Chemistry and Hair Mineral Analysis.* CJ Frompovich Publications, 1983.

Gibson, Douglas. *Studies of Homeopathic Remedies.* Beaconsfield Publishers, Bucks, England, 1987.

Gittleman, Ann Louise. *Guess What Came to Dinner: Parasites and Your Health.* Avery Pub Group, Garden City Park, NY, 1993.

Hamilton, Kirk. *Clinical Pearls in Nutrition and Preventive Medicine.* ITServices, Sacramento, CA, 1993.

Heinerman, John. *Science of Herbal Medicine.* Bi-World Publishers, Orem, Utah, 1980.

Huggins, Hal A, DDS, MS. *Its All In Your Head.* Paragon Press, Honesdale, PA, 1993.

Krohn, Jacqueline, MD. *Allergy Relief & Prevention.* Hartley & Marks, Point Roberts, WA, 1991.

Kuzemko, Jan. *Is Your Child Allergic? A Practical Guide for Parents.* Thorsons Publishers, Northamptonshire, England, 1988.

Lieberman, Shari, and Bruning, Nancy. *The Real Vitamin & Mineral Book.* Avery Pub Co, Garden City Park, NY, 1990.

Miller, Neil Z. *Vaccines: Are They Really Safe and Effective?* New Atlantean Press, Santa Fe, NM, 1994.

Murray, Michael, ND, and Pizzorno, Joseph, ND. *Encyclopedia of Natural Medicine.* Prima Publishing, Rocklin, CA, 1990.

Priest, AW, and Priest, LR. *Herbal Medication.* Fowler & Co, Exxex, England, 1982.

Ritchason, Jack, ND. *Vitamin and Health Encyclopedia.* Woodland Publishing, Pleasant Grove, UT, 1996.

Ritchason, Jack, ND. *The Little Herb Encyclopedia.* Woodland Publishing, Pleasant Grove, UT, 1995.

Rimington, Dennis W, MD. Higa, Barbara W, RD, *Back to Health - A Comprehensive Medical and Nutritional Yeast Control Program.* Vitality House International, Provo, Utah, 1989.

Santillo, Humbart, BS, MH, *Natural Healing with Herbs.* Hohm Press, Prescott Valley, AZ, 1984.

Smith, Lendon H., MD. *Feed Your Body Right.* M Evans & Co, NY, NY, 1994.

Smith, Trevor. *The Homeopathic Treatment of Emotional Illness.* Thorsons Publishers, NY, NY, 9184.

Somer, Elizabeth, MA, RD. *The Essential Guide to Vitamins and Minerals.* Harper Collins, NY, NY, 1992.

Spoerke, David G. *Herbal Medications.* Woodgridge Press Publishing Co, Santa Barbara, CA, 1980.

Stanway, Penny. *Foods for Common Ailments - How to Use Everyday Foods to Prevent and Treat 80 Common Health Problems.* Simon & Schuster, NY, NY, 1989.

Tenney, Louise. *Today's Herbal Health for Children.* Woodland Publishing, Pleasant Grove Utah, 1996.

Trattler, Ross, ND. *Better Health, Natural Healing - How to Get Well Without Drugs or Surgery.* McGraw-Hill Book Co, NY, NY, 1985.

Weil, Andrew, MD. *Natural Health, Natural Medicine.* Houghton Mifflin Co, Boston, Mass, 1990.

Weintraub, Skye, ND. *Minding Your Body.* Complementary Medicine Publishing Co, Portland, OR, 1995.

Weintraub, Skye, ND. *Natural Healing with Cell Salts.* Woodland Publishing, Pleasant Grove, UT, 1996.

Wright, Jonathan V, MD. *Dr. Wright's Guide to Healing with Nutrition.* Keats Publishing, New Canaan, CT, 1990.

RECOMMENDED READING

Allergies and Your Family, by Doris J. Rapp. Sterling Publishing Co, NY.
Allergies and the Hyperactive Child, by Doris J. Rapp. Sovereign Books, NY.
Allergy Recipes, by Sally Rockwell. Nutrition Survival Press, 4703 Stone Way N, Seattle, WA 98103. Recipes easily prepared with or without gluten, grains, peanuts, soy, milk products, eggs, yeast and refined sugars. Recipes listed in a rotation-diet format.

The American Vegetarian Cookbook, by Marilyn Diamond. From *The Fit For Life Kitchen* series, Warner Books, Inc. Has a section on substitutions for commonly found ingredients. There are dairy-free recipes and other ways to replace animal products in recipes.

An Illustrated Guide to Organic Gardening and *How to Garden in Harmony with Nature*. Sunset Publishing Corp, Manol Park, CA 94025.

Are You Allergic, by William G. Crook. Professional Books, Jackson, TN.

Baking with Amaranth, by Marge Jones. Illinois Amaranth Company, Box 464 R, Mundelein, IL 60060. A recipe booklet with ways to use this nutty flavored food. Contains no dairy products or wheat in the tasty recipes. You can even order the grain from the Illinois Amaranth Co.

Behavioral Problems of Children: Some Causes; Some Solutions, by Jane Hersey. Pear Tree Press, PO Box 30146, Alexandria, VA 22310.

Brain Allergies, by William H. Philpott and Dwight K. Kalita. Keats Publishing, Inc, New Cannaan, CT 06840.

Cookbook/ Guide to Eating for Allergies, by Virginia Nichols. 3550 Fair Oaks Drive, Xenia, OH 45385. Information on food families.

The Cure is in the Kitchen, by Sherry A. Rogers, MD. Prestige Publishing, (315) 455-7012. Covers case studies of patients with chronic diseases, ranging from rheumatoid arthritis to multiple chemical sensitivities, focusing on the switch to macrobiotic lifestyles and the subsequent recoveries.

Diet For a Poisoned Planet, by David Steinman. Ballantine Books. This book has additional resources in the appendixes for organic food mail-order shopping. It also has many other helpful resources.

Environmental Hazards in Your School, A resource handbook. United States Environmental Protection Agency (EPA), Publication #2DT-2001

Environmental Poisons in Our Food, by J. Gordon Millichap, MD. PNB Publishers, Box 11391, Chicago, IL 60611.

The Neurotoxicity of Food Additives, Health Press, PO Drawer 1388, Santa Fe, NM 87504.

Help for the Hyperactive Child, by William G. Crook. Professional Books, Inc, 681 Skyline Dr., Jackson, TN 38301.

The Impossible Child (in School, at Home). The Practical Allergy Research Foundation, PO Box 60, Buffalo, NY 14223-0060.

Is This Your Child? by Doris J. Rapp. William Morrow and Company, Inc, NY.

Is Your Child Hyperactive? by Benjamin Feingold, MD. Explores how nutrition is related to the behavior of children.

Off to School with Food Allergies: A Guide for Parents and Teachers. Send $8.00 plus $1.00 for shipping and handling to The Food Allergy Network, 4744 Holly Avenue, Fairfax, VA 22030-5647. The guide is packed with suggestions for communicating the needs of the child to school officials. Included are lunch tips and answers to frequently asked questions about food allergies.

1995 National Organic Directory, Box 464, Davis, CA 95617. (800) 852-3832 or (916) 756-8518. This is a comprehensive guide to organic farmers and wholesalers who sell mail-order foods to consumers. The guide is fully indexed and lists over 140 suppliers by commodity, state, and company. You can find organic suppliers for everything from artichokes and azuki beans to pheasant and wine. The directory is available for $34.95 plus $5.50 first-class shipping and handling.

The Natural Way to Control Hyperactivity. Watercress Press, San Antonio, TX.

Staying Well in a Toxic World, by Lynn Lawson. The Noble Press, Inc, 213 W Institute Place, Suite 508, Chicago, IL 60610. Lawson writes from first-hand experience of how chronic illnesses can result from toxic chemical exposure. This book defines the problem and offers valuable recommendations for avoidance or minimizing exposures. She currently coordinates the Chicago area multiple chemical sensitivity support group.

Tracking Down Hidden Food Allergy, by William G. Crook, MD. Professional Books, PO Box 3494, Jackson, TN 38301. Cleverly illustrated, easy-to-follow instructions to help you carry out elimination diets. It contains other sources of foods, shopping tips, menus, and recipes to help manage food sensitivities.

Tired or Toxic, by Dr. Sherry Rogers, MD. Prestige Publishers, Box 3161, Syracuse, NY 13220. (800) 846-6687 or (315) 455-7862.

Wellness Against All Odds, by Dr. Sherry Rogers, MD. Prestige Publishing, PO Box 3161, Syracuse, NY 13220. (800) 846-6687 or (315) 455-7862.

The Yeast Connection Cookbook, by William G. Crook and Marjorie Hurt Jones. MAST Enterprises, 2615 N Fourth Ave, Coeur d'Alene, ID 83814. This book contains recipes that go along with a yeast-free diet.

The Asthma and Allergy Foundation of America has developed a special food-allergy support group. Questions and requests to form your own support group should be directed to Nancy Sanker, (303) 221-9165, 1412 Miramont Dr, Fort Collins, CO 80524. Every affiliated group will receive a special food-allergy library pack to serve as the base of the group lending library. It includes one copy of each of the four following books. Her other books and newsletter are also available:

The Complete Book of Children's Allergies, by B. Robert Feldman, MD.

The Food Allergy Cookbook, and *Food Allergy: A Primer for People,* by Anne Munoz-Furlong.

A Nutrition Guide to Food Allergies, by S. Allen Bock, MD.

BOOKS FOR CHILDREN AND TEENS

Jumpin' Johnny, Get Back to Work! A Child's Guide to ADHD and Hyperactivity, by M. Gordon. GSI Publications, DeWitt, NY, 1991. For ages 7-12.

Learning Disabilities and the Don't Give Up Kid, Verbal Images Press, Fairport, NY, 1990. For classmates and children with learning disabilities and attention difficulties, ages 7-12.

Learning to Slow Down and Pay Attention, by K. Nadeau and E. Dixon. Chesapeake Psychological Publications, Annandale, VA, 1993.

Living with a Brother or Sister with Special Needs: A Book for Sibs, by D. Meyer, P. Vadasy, and R. Fewell. University of Washington Press, Seattle, 1985.

My Brother Matthew, by M. Thompson. Woodbine House, Rockville, MD, 1992.

Otto Learns about his Medication, by M Galvin. Magination Press, NY, 1988. For young children.

Putting on the Brakes: Young People's Guide to Understanding Attention Deficit Hyperactivity Disorder, by P. Quinn & J. Stern.Magination Press, New York, 1991. For ages 8-12.

Shelly the Hyperactive Turtle, by D. Moss. Woodbine House, Rockville MD, 1989. For young children.

BOOKS FOR TEACHERS

Attention Deficit Hyperactivity Disorder. R. Barkley, Guilford Publications, NY, 1990. Four 40-minute videocassettes in VHS format.

Attention Without Tension: A Teacher's Handbook on Attention Disorders. E. Copeland, E, and V. Love. 3 C's of Childhood, Atlanta, GA, 1992.

I Can't Sit Still-Educating and Affirming Inattentive and Hyperactive Children. D. Johnson, ETR Associates, Santa Cruz, CA, 1992. Contains suggestions for parents, teachers, and other care providers of children to age 10.

Off to School with Food Allergies: A Guide for Parents and Teachers. The Food Allergy Network, 4744 Holly Avenue, Fairfax, VA, 22030-5647. Send $8.00 plus $1.00 for shipping and handling. The guide includes information about food allergies, strategies for reducing the risk of allergic reactions in the classroom, and a checklist of key questions to ask parents. It also includes a medical form to be filled out by the student's doctor.

The ADD Hyperactivity Handbook for Schools, H. Parker, Impact Publications, Plantation, FL, 1992.

BOOKS FOR PARENTS

A Parent's Guide to Attention Deficit Disorders. L Bain, Dell Publishing NY, 1991.

Attention Deficit Hyperactivity Disorder: Questions & Answers for Parents. G. Greenberg, S. Horn, and F. Wade, Research Press, Champaign, IL, 1991.

Attention, Please! A Comprehensive Guide for Successfully Parenting Children with Attention Disorders and Hyperactivity. E. Copeland, and V. Love, SPI Press, Atlanta, GA, 1991.

Coping with ADD. Mary Ellen Beugin, Detselig Enterprises, Calgary, Alberta, 1990.

Creating Your Personal Vision—A Mind-Body Guide For Better Eyesight, Dr. Samuel A. Berne, Behavioral Optometrist. Color Stone Press, 1300 Luisa St., #4, Santa Fe, New Mexico 87505, (505) 820-2527.

Defiant Children. R. Barkley, Guilford Press, NY, 1987.

Discipline: A Sourcebook of 50 Failsafe Techniques for Parents. J. Windell, New York: Collier Books, 1991.

Hyperactivity: Why Won't My Child Pay Attention? S. Goldstein, and M. Goldstein, J. Wiley, NY, 1992.

Maybe You Know My Kid: A Parent's Guide to Identifying, Understanding, and Helping your Child with ADHD. M. Fowler, Birch Lane Press, NY, 1990.

Negotiating the Special Education Maze: A Guide for Parents and Teachers (2d ed). W. Anderson, S. Chitwood, S, and D Hayden, Woodbine House, Rockville, MD, 1990.

Optimizing Special Education: How Parents Can Make a Difference. N. Wilson, Insight Books, NY, 1992.

Why Johnnie Can't Concentrate - Coping with Attention Deficit Problems. Robert A. Moss, Bantam, 1990.

OTHER RESOURCES

For individuals with a computer and modem, there are on-line bulletin boards where parents, and medical professionals share experiences, offer emotional support, and ask and respond to questions. Two such on-line services include CompuServe (800) 848-8990 and America Online (800) 827-6364. You may also wish to check with other national and local on-line communications companies to see if they offer similar services. The internet has many sources of information about ADD.

RELATED MATERIALS

Attention Deficit Disorder Information Packet and *Know Your Brain Fact Sheet*
are both available from NIH Neurological Institute, P.O. Box 5801,
Bethesda, MD 20824, (800) 352-9424.

Learning Disabilities (NIH Pub. No. 93-3611) and *Plain Talk about
Depression* (NIH Pub. No. 93-3561). These are available by contacting:
NIMH, Room 7C-02, 5600 Fishers Lane, Rockville, MD 20857.

INDEX

DATE DUE

		ILL	
	DEC 1 0 2003		
	NOV 1 8 2004		
APR 2 1 2005			
	APR 1 9 2007		
APR 2 5 2008			
	NOV 2 3 2013		

Demco, Inc. 38-293